ABC of Prostate Cancer

EDITED BY

Prokar Dasgupta
Consultant Urological Surgeon
Department of Urology
King's College London
Guy's and St Thomas' Hospital NHS Foundation Trust
London, UK

Roger S. Kirby
Consultant Urologist
The Prostate Centre, London, UK

Foreword by Peter T. Scardino

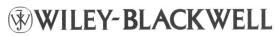
WILEY-BLACKWELL
A John Wiley & Sons, Ltd., Publication

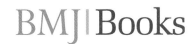
BMJ|Books

This edition first published 2012 © 2012 by Blackwell Publishing Ltd.

Blackwell Publishing was acquired by John Wiley & Sons in February 2007. Blackwell's publishing program has been merged with Wiley's global Scientific, Technical and Medical business to form Wiley-Blackwell.

Registered office: John Wiley & Sons Ltd, The Atrium, Southern Gate, Chichester, West Sussex, PO19 8SQ, UK

Editorial offices: 9600 Garsington Road, Oxford, OX4 2DQ, UK

       The Atrium, Southern Gate, Chichester, West Sussex, PO19 8SQ, UK

       111 River Street, Hoboken, NJ 07030-5774, USA

For details of our global editorial offices, for customer services and for information about how to apply for permission to reuse the copyright material in this book please see our website at www.wiley.com/wiley-blackwell

Library of Congress Cataloging-in-Publication Data

ABC of prostate cancer / edited by Prokar Dasgupta, Roger S. Kirby ; foreword by Peter T. Scardino. – 1st ed.
   p. ; cm. -- (ABC series)
  Includes bibliographical references and index.
  ISBN-13: 978-1-4443-3437-1 (pbk. : alk. paper) ISBN-10: 1-4443-3437-9 (pbk. : alk. paper)
  1. Prostate – Cancer. I. Dasgupta, Prokar. II. Kirby, R. S. (Roger S.) III. Series: ABC series (Malden, Mass.).
  [DNLM: 1. Prostatic Neoplasms. WJ 762]
  RC280.P7A23 2012
  616.99'463 – dc23

                2011015319

A catalogue record for this book is available from the British Library.

This book is published in the following electronic formats: ePDF 9781444346909; ePub 9781444346916; Mobi 9781444346923

Set in 9.25/12 Minion by Laserwords Private Limited, Chennai, India
Printed in Singapore by Ho Printing Singapore Pte Ltd

1   2012

ABC of
Prostate Cancer

ABC series

An outstanding collection of resources – written by specialists for non-specialists

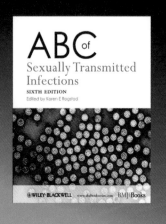

ABC of Sexually Transmitted Infections
SIXTH EDITION
Edited by Karen E Rogstad

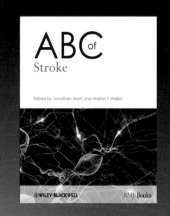

ABC of Stroke
Edited by Jonathan Mant and Marion F Walker

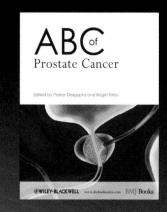

ABC of Prostate Cancer
Edited by Prokar Dasgupta and Roger Kirby

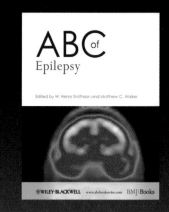

ABC of Epilepsy
Edited by W. Henry Smithson and Matthew C. Walker

The *ABC* series contains a wealth of indispensable resources for GPs, GP registrars, junior doctors, doctors in training and all those in primary care

▶ **Now fully revised and updated**
▶ **Highly illustrated, informative and a practical source of knowledge**
▶ **An easy-to-use resource, covering the symptoms, investigations, treatment and management of conditions presenting in day-to-day practice and patient support**
▶ **Full colour photographs and illustrations aid diagnosis and patient understanding of a condition**

For more information on all books in the *ABC* series, including links to further information, references and links to the latest official guidelines, please visit:

www.abcbookseries.com

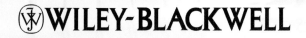

WILEY-BLACKWELL

BMJ|Books

Contents

Contributors

Peter Acher
Specialist Registrar in Urology, Guy's and St Thomas' Hospital NHS Foundation Trust, London, UK

Hashim U. Ahmed
MRC Fellow in Uro-oncology and Clinical Lecturer in Urology, Division of Surgery and Interventional Sciences, University College Hospital London, London, UK

Richard J. Bryant
NIHR Clinical Lecturer in Urology, Nuffield Department of Surgical Sciences, University of Oxford, Oxford, UK

Declan Cahill
Consultant Urological Surgeon, Guy's and St Thomas' Hospital NHS Foundation Trust, London, UK

Ben Challacombe
Consultant Urological Surgeon, Guy's and St Thomas' Hospital NHS Foundation Trust, London, UK

Ashish Chandra
Consultant Pathologist, Guy's and St Thomas' Hospital NHS Foundation Trust, London, UK

Anthony J. Costello
Professorial Fellow, Department of Urology, The Royal Melbourne Hospital, The Peter MacCallum Cancer Centre, Melbourne, VIC, Australia

Prokar Dasgupta
Consultant Urological Surgeon, Department of Urology, King's College London, Guy's and St Thomas' Hospital NHS Foundation Trust, London, UK

Reena Davda
Specialist Registrar in Clinical Oncology, University College Hospital London, London, UK

John Davies
Consultant Urological Surgeon, University of Surrey, Guildford, UK

Louise Dickinson
Clinical Research Fellow in Urology, Division of Surgery and Interventional Sciences, University College Hospital London, London, UK

Judith Dockray
King's College London, London, UK

Oussama Elhage
Medical Research Council Centre for Transplantation, King's College London, London, UK

Mark Emberton
Professor of Interventional Oncology, University College London and Honorary Consultant Urological Surgeon, University College Hospital London, London, UK

Mark R. Feneley
Consultant Urologist, University College Hospital London, London, UK

John M. Fitzpatrick
Professor of Surgery, UCD School of Medicine and Medical Science, Mater Misericordiae University Hospital, University College Dublin, Dublin, Ireland

Christine Galustian
King's College London, London, UK

James Halls
Specialist Registrar Radiology, Department of Radiology, St George's Healthcare NHS Trust, London, UK

Freddie C. Hamdy
Nuffield Professor of Surgery, Professor of Urology and Head, Nuffield Department of Surgical Sciences, University of Oxford, Oxford, UK

Wim van Haute
Urological Surgeon, Department of Urology, St Rembert Hospital, Torhout; St Jan Hospital, Bruges, Belgium

Alastair Henderson
Consultant Urological Surgeon, Maidstone and Tunbridge Wells NHS Trust, Maidstone, UK

Lars Holmberg
Professor of Cancer Epidemiology, Division of Cancer Studies, Medical School, King's College London, London, UK

Roger S. Kirby
Consultant Urologist, The Prostate Centre, London, UK

Pardeep Kumar
Specialist Registrar in Urology and Intuitive Fellow in Robotics, Guy's and St Thomas' Hospital NHS Foundation Trust, London, UK

David Landau
Consultant Clinical Oncologist, Guy's and St Thomas' Hospital NHS Foundation Trust, London, UK

Gordon Muir
King's College London, London, UK

Declan G. Murphy
Uro-Oncologist, The Peter MacCallum Cancer Centre, Associate Professor of Urology, University of Melbourne, Melbourne, VIC, Australia

Uday Patel
Consultant Radiologist, Department of Radiology, St George's Healthcare NHS Trust, London, UK

Heather Payne
Consultant in Clinical Oncology, University College Hospital London, London, UK

Jim Peabody
Attending Urologist and Fellowship Director at Henry Ford Health System, Henry Ford Hospital, Detroit, MI, USA

Rick Popert
Department of Urology, Guy's and St Thomas' Hospital NHS Foundation Trust, London, UK

Hein van Poppel
Full Professor of Urology, Katholieke Universiteit, Chairman Department of Urology, University Hospital Gasthuisberg, Leuven, Belgium

Asad Qureshi
Clinical Fellow in Clinical Oncology, Guy's and St Thomas' Hospital NHS Foundation Trust, London, UK

Megan S. Schober
Department of Urology, William Beaumont School of Medicine at Oakland University, Royal Oak, MI, USA

Karl-Dietrich Sievert
Professor of Urology, Director, Uro-oncology, Neurourology, Incontinence and Reconstructive Urology, Department of Urology, University of Tübingen, Tübingen, Germany

Richard Smith
Medical Research Council Centre for Transplantation, King's College London, London, UK

Prasanna Sooriakumaran
Visiting Fellow in Urology, Robotic Prostatectomy and Urologic Oncology Outcomes, James Buchanan Brady Foundation Department of Urology, Weill Cornell Medical College, New York Presbyterian Hospital, New York, NY, USA

Abhishek Srivastava
Research Associate, Robotic Prostatectomy and Urologic Oncology Outcomes, James Buchanan Brady Foundation Department of Urology, Weill Cornell Medical College, New York Presbyterian Hospital, New York, NY, USA

Ashutosh Tewari
Ronald P. Lynch Professor of Urology, Director- LeFrak Center for Robotics, Director- Prostate Cancer Institute, James Buchanan Brady Foundation Department of Urology, Weill Cornell Medical College, New York Presbyterian Hospital, New York, NY, USA

Murali Varma
Consultant Histopathologist, University Hospital of Wales, Cardiff, UK

Nadia Walsh
Superintendent Planning Radiographer, Guy's and St. Thomas' Hospital NHS Foundation Trust, London, UK

R. William G. Watson
Associate Professor of Cancer Biology, UCD School of Medicine and Medical Science, Conway Institute of Biomolecular and Biomedical Research, University College Dublin, Dublin, Ireland

Robin Weston
Department of Urology, The Royal Melbourne Hospital, The Peter MacCallum Cancer Centre, The Australian Prostate Cancer Research Centre, Epworth Richmond Hospital, Melbourne, VIC, Australia

Foreword

Men diagnosed with prostate cancer, and the physicians who care for them, are faced with a wealth of information about this disease, including a variety of treatment options. Conflicting expert opinions make it especially difficult to choose with confidence the right treatment at the right time. This new edition of the ABC series, "ABC of Prostate Cancer," provides a clear, comprehensive, up-to-date overview of all aspects of the diagnosis and treatment of prostate cancer. It might have been called "Prostate Cancer from A to Z." In essence, it is a collection of chapters by world renowned experts in the field. Clearly written, comprehensive yet concise, and beautifully illustrated, this volume will provide a good starting point for physicians and medical personnel who are not experts in prostate cancer. The volume is thorough and covers virtually every aspect of prostate cancer treatment. The chapters on new treatment approaches are particularly impressive.

We are living through a revolutionary time in the development of systemic therapy for prostate cancer, including hormonally active agents such as abiraterone and MDV3100, the new antiandrogen produced by Charles Sawyers and developed by the Medivation. The first vaccine for prostate cancer approved by the United States FDA, sipuleucel-T, has launched a new era in the immunotherapy of cancer. This volume describes those advances and recently approved systemic chemotherapy drugs in detail. For localized prostate cancer, the chapters on robotic assisted laparoscopic prostatectomy and on focal therapy, an unproven yet highly attractive approach now undergoing testing in clinical trials, are well presented.

The reader should be cautioned, however, that these chapters represent the optimistic view of experts who are advocates for the diagnostic or treatment approach that they describe. The chapters do not represent the consensus of a multidisciplinary panel of experts. That makes this book an excellent place to start when one is interested in a concise, state-of-the-art overview of each approach, but more information would be necessary before a final, informed decision should be made.

As the author of a book on prostate cancer for the layman and a practicing physician myself, I often point out to patients that prostate cancer is a condition that warrants a second or even third opinion from experts across the fields of urology, medical oncology and radiation oncology before a final decision is reached. A thoughtful patient is wise to ask his personal physician to help digest the sometimes contradictory opinions offered by specialists. Those of us within the field of prostate cancer know that how well a treatment is delivered is as important as which treatment one chooses, so experience and expertise in the chosen treatment is crucial to realizing the best outcome.

The medical community should welcome this new approach to providing comprehensive yet concise information about the state of the art for prostate cancer. The authors of these chapters and the editors who organized this new text should be congratulated. This is a fine place to begin to learn about one of the more complicated and controversial diseases that men face.

Peter T. Scardino, MD
The David H. Koch Chair
Chairman, Department of Surgery
Memorial Sloan-Kettering Cancer Center
New York, NY, USA

CHAPTER 1

Applied Anatomy of the Prostate

Prasanna Sooriakumaran[1], *Karl-Dietrich Sievert*[2], *Abhishek Srivastava*[1]
and Ashutosh Tewari[1]

[1]Prostate Cancer Institute and Lefrak Center of Robotic Surgery, James Buchanan Brady Foundation Department of Urology,
Weill Cornell Medical College, New York Presbyterian Hospital, New York, NY, USA
[2]Department of Urology, University of Tübingen, Tübingen, Germany

---

OVERVIEW

- The prostate is composed of four zones: transitional, central, peripheral, and anterior fibromuscular stroma
- The ejaculatory ducts open into the prostatic urethra on either side of the verumontanum
- The external urethral sphincter (both voluntary and involuntary elements) lies immediately distal to the verumontanum while the internal urethral sphincter (involuntary) lies at the bladder neck
- The prostate lies in a hammock of nerves which can be divided into three zones: proximal neurovascular plate, predominant neurovascular bundles, and accessory distal neural pathways Cavernous nerves exceed the posterolateral track and distribute in a more widespread range from anterolateral to posterior of the gland
- The prostate is surrounded by prostatic fascia andendopelvic fascia, with Denonvillier's fascia separating it from the fascia propria of the rectum

---

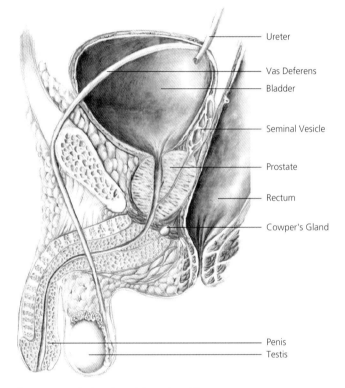

Figure 1.1 Sagittal section of the male pelvis.

The basic anatomy

The prostate gland develops after puberty as a result of the testosterone surge. It reaches a size of 20cc in the normal adult, measuring 3 cm in length, 4 cm in width, and 2 cm in depth. Its size and shape can be approximated to that of a walnut. It is located at the base of the bladder, where it surrounds the proximal urethra. In this position, it lies above the urogenital diaphragm between the rectum and the symphysis pubis (Figure 1.1). It is described as having anterior, posterior, and lateral surfaces. Its base is contiguous with the bladder and its apex narrows inferiorly. There is no 'true' capsule to the prostate, but rather a 'false' capsule of fibromuscular stroma which disappears towards the apex of the gland. The prostate is surrounded by fascial structures (Figure 1.2) anteriorly and anterolaterally by the prostatic fascia, and posteriorly by Denonvillier's

fascia which separates it from the fascia propria of the rectum. Laterally, the prostatic fascia merges with the endopelvic fascia (also called the lateral pelvic or levator fascia). The prostatic base is covered with a posterior layer of detrusor apron from the bladder muscle. Abutting the prostate posteriorly are the seminal vesicles and vasa (ducti) deferentia (Figure 1.3).

The prostate gland itself is composed of ducts and alveoli that are lined by tall columnar epithelium (70%) within a stroma of fibromuscular tissue (30%). The urethra does not run straight through the middle of the gland as is the common medical student misconception, but rather takes a curved course, running anteriorly as it proceeds from proximal to distal, such that it ends up close to the prostate's anterior surface. It is lined by transitional epithelium

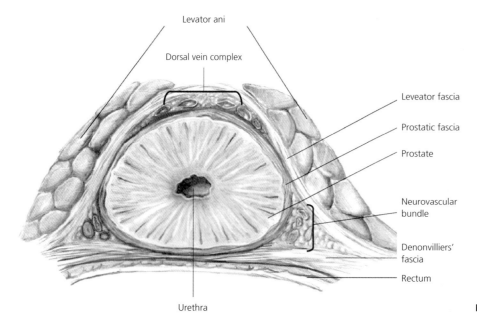

Levator ani

Dorsal vein complex

Leveator fascia

Prostatic fascia

Prostate

Neurovascular bundle

Denonvilliers' fascia

Rectum

Urethra

Figure 1.2 Fascial relations of the prostate.

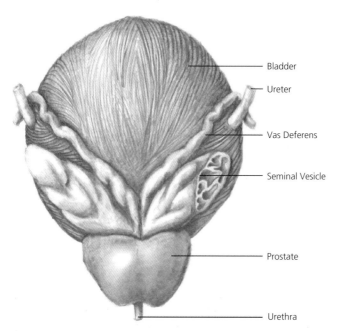

Bladder

Ureter

Vas Deferens

Seminal Vesicle

Prostate

Urethra

Figure 1.3 The posterior relations of the prostate.

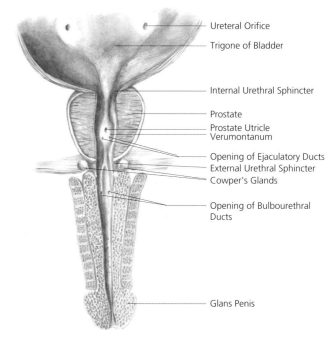

Ureteral Orifice

Trigone of Bladder

Internal Urethral Sphincter

Prostate

Prostate Utricle
Verumontanum

Opening of Ejaculatory Ducts
External Urethral Sphincter
Cowper's Glands

Opening of Bulbourethral Ducts

Glans Penis

Figure 1.4 Cross-sectional anatomy of the male lower urinary tract.

throughout most of its length, and squamous epithelium at its distal end, hence, cancer of the urethra is either transitional cell or squamous cell carcinoma, and not adenocarcinoma as for the prostate. Those urothelial cancers are highly aggressive. A urethral crest runs the length of the prostate and disappears in the striated external urethral sphincter (rhabdosphincter). The prostatic sinuses run alongside the crest and all the prostatic glands discharge into this. The small slit of the prostatic utricle is found on the verumontanum (colliculus). The ejaculatory ducts open just lateral to the verumontanum and this is where the seminal vesicle contents are discharged (via the vasa) during emission (Figure 1.4). This allows the seminal fluid to mix with the prostatic secretions such that the final ejaculate is a mixture of these two components.

Just proximal to the verumontanum is the external urethral sphincter (EUS) which is a horseshoe-shaped structure which surrounds the prostatic apex craniodorsolaterally, is deficient posteriorly, and has both striated (voluntary) and smooth muscle (involuntary) components. Hence, during a transurethral resection of the prostate (TURP) for benign prostatic enlargement (BPE), the verumontanum serves as the limit for proximal resection so that the EUS is not damaged. The internal urethral sphincter is located at the bladder neck where the prostato-vesical junction is, and is purely under involuntary control (hence, it is composed of smooth muscle). It not only completes the continence mechanism but also makes antegrade ejaculation possible. The internal urethral sphincter is invariably damaged during a TURP so that, were the EUS to also be damaged, then urinary incontinence would be inevitable. This is why the verumontanum (or 'veru' to those that know it well) is such an important landmark during TURP.

Lymphovascular supply

The arterial supply to the prostate arises from the inferior vesical artery (itself a branch of the internal iliac artery). As the inferior vesical artery approaches the prostate gland, it becomes the prostatic artery. This then divides into two main groups of arteries: the urethral group and the capsular group. The urethral arteries penetrate the prostato-vesical junction posterolaterally and travel inward, perpendicular to the urethra. They approach the bladder neck in the 1- to-5 o'clock and 7- to-11 o'clock positions, with the largest branches located posteriorly. The capsular artery gives off a few small branches to the false capsule of the prostate, but, in the main, runs posterolaterally to the prostate along with the cavernous nerves (to form the so-called neurovascular bundle), before ending at the urogenital diaphragm.

The venous drainage of the prostate is via the periprostatic plexus of veins to both the dorsal venous complex (of Santorini) superiorly and the inferior vesical vein to the hypogastric vein. These then both drain into the internal iliac vein. The dorsal venous complex (DVC) lies over the anterior aspect of the prostate and is the commonest source of bleeding during a radical prostatectomy. Just lateral to the DVC are the puboprostatic ligaments (PPL) which are condensations of the endopelvic fascia and attach the prostate to the pubic symphysis. The PPL may be important in maintaining continence, and are thus often spared during radical prostatectomy.

As is true of much human anatomy, the lymphatic drainage of the prostate follows that of the veins. Hence, for the prostate, this is to the obturator and hypogastric nodes, and then on to the internal iliac and aortic nodes. It is important to note, however, that prostatic lymphatic drainage is not always predictable in a stepwise manner, and 25% of cases of prostate cancer drain directly to nodes outside the pelvis (internal iliac or higher), making the extent of pelvic lymphadenectomy in high-risk prostate cancer a subject of much debate.

Zonal anatomy

Throughout the nineteenth century, the prostate was described as having two lobes, with each lobe having its own ducts. In 1906, Howe described a middle (or median) lobe. In 1912, Lowsley described five lobes: two lateral lobes, a posterior lobe, the middle lobe, and an atrophied embryological anterior lobe. However, these lobes were visible only in BPE and not the normal prostate. This lobar concept thus left much to be desired, and in 1968, McNeal replaced it with his concentric zones concept (Figure 1.5).

The transition zone consists of 5–10% of the glandular tissue of the prostate and is responsible for most of the BPE that affects the prostates of older men. The prostatic ducts lead into the junction of the pre-prostatic and prostatic urethra, and travel on the posterolateral aspects of the EUS.

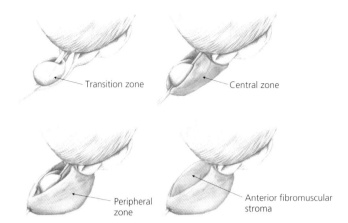

Figure 1.5 McNeal's zones of the prostate.

The ducts of the central zone arise circumferentially around the openings of the ejaculatory ducts. These glands are histologically distinct and appear to be Wolffian (mesonephric) in embryological origin. Only 1–2% of prostate cancers arise from this zone.

The peripheral zone makes up 60% of the prostatic volume. Its ducts drain into the prostatic sinus along the entire length. Some 70% of carcinomas arise from this zone which is also commonly affected by prostatitis (hence, prostatitis and cancer can co-exist in men).

The anterior fibromuscular stroma makes up approximately 30% of the gland, and extends from the bladder neck to the EUS anteriorly. It is compressed in BPE and rarely involved in prostate cancer, though anterior cancers should be suspected when repeat conventional prostatic biopsies which do not sample the anterior aspects well come back negative; hence, the use of saturation or template biopsies to sample these anterior aspects.

Neuroanatomy

Using dissections of male fetuses and newborn cadavers, Walsh and Donker first demonstrated the course of the cavernous nerve (the main nerve responsible for erectile function). This led to the concept of the macroscopic neurovascular bundle (NVB) that is located between the endopelvic and prostatic fasciae and runs along the posterolateral aspect of the prostate until it enters the urogenital diaphragm. However, recently, there have been observations that refute the dogma that the cavernous nerve is always within the NVB. Using intraoperative electrical stimulation with simultaneous measurement of intracavernosal pressure, our group, as well as others, discovered that the distribution of cavernous nerves was wider than that of the neurovascular bundle. Our group described the distribution of these nerves and they can be thought of as forming three broad zones: the trizonal concept.

The first zone is the proximal neurovascular plate (PNP) which is located lateral to the bladder neck, seminal vesicles, and branches of the inferior vesical vessels. Proximally, the PNP is derived from the pelvic (inferior hypogastric) plexus and cavernous nerves run in its most distal part. It is not only composed of parasympathetic nerves as commonly thought, but also has sympathetic contributions from

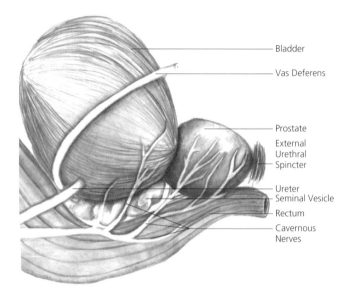

- Bladder
- Vas Deferens
- Prostate
- External Urethral Spinter
- Ureter
- Seminal Vesicle
- Rectum
- Cavernous Nerves

Figure 1.6 Anatomy of the cavernous nerves.

the hypogastric nerve. The second zone is the predominant neurovascular bundle (PNB) which corresponds with the classical NVB. The PNB is located between the endopelvic and prostatic fasciae at the posterolateral aspect of the prostate (the same as the NVB). The third zone is the accessory distal neural pathways (ANP). These smaller accessories off the PNB travel in the prostatic and Denonvillier's fasciae, and may serve as additional conduits for neural impulses to both the cavernous tissues and the EUS. The ANP can cross from one side to the other, and thus may also serve as a safety mechanism to provide back-up neural cross-talk between the two sides.

The prostate can be thought of as lying within a hammock of these nerves, so that the neural zones surround the majority of the gland. This concept is then very different to the conventional concept wherein the prostate lies between two NVBs that course its posterolateral aspects like train tracks.

Recent results show that the posterolateral accumulation of nerves (the NVB) is supplemented by additional main localisations in the anterior mid-part of the prostate and, even more so, on the posterior surface of the prostatic apex. The main extra-capsular prostatic nerves expand from the base to the mid of the prostate before they narrow in the posterolateral and posterior sectors around the prostate. The extent of these additional localisations of nerves seems to vary from individual to individual.

There is evidence for clear differences between the main localisations of nerve qualities along the prostate. Currently the consensus opinion for the most likely localisation of the nerve fibres responsible for erectile functionality is the posterior margin of the NVB. Recent studies provide a differential mapping of nerves of different characteristics. The localisations of cavernous nerves considerably seem to exceed the course of the posterolateral NVB both in the anterior and, to an even greater extent, in the posterior direction, resulting in a main localisation of erectile nerve fibres along an oblique shape in a base-lateral towards postero-apical track around the prostate (Figure 1.6).

Further reading

Sievert KD, Hennenlotter J, Laible I, Amend B, Schilling D, Anastasiadis A, et al. The periprostatic autonomic nerves: bundle or layer? *Eur Urol* 2008;**54**(5):1109–16.

Takenaka A, Tewari A, Hara A, Leung RA, Kurokawa K, Murakami G, et al. Pelvic autonomic nerve mapping around the prostate by intraoperative electrical stimulation with simultaneous measurement of intracavernous and intraurethral pressure. *J Urol* 2007;**177**(1):225–9.

Tewari A, Peabody JO, Fischer M, Sarle R, Vallencien G, Delmas V, et al. An operative and anatomic study to help in nerve sparing during laparoscopic and robotic radical prostatectomy. *Eur Urol* 2003;**43**(5):444–54.

Tewari A, Takenaka A, Mtui E, Horninger W, Peschel R, Bartsch G, Vaughan ED. The proximal neurovascular plate and tri-zonal neural architecture around the prostate gland: importance in the athermal robotic technique of nerve-sparing prostatectomy. *BJU Int* 2006;**98**(2):314–23.

Walz J, Burnett AL, Costello AJ, Eastham JA, Graefen M, Guillonneau B, et al. A critical analysis of the current knowledge of surgical anatomy related to optimization of cancer control and preservation of continence and erection in candidates for radical prostatectomy. *Eur Urol* 2010;**57**(2):179–92.

Acknowledgements/Disclosures

Prasanna Sooriakumaran is the ACMI Corp. Endourological Society Fellow 2010–2011, and also receives financial support from Prostate UK.

A.K.T. discloses that he is the principal investigator on research grants from Intuitive Surgical Inc. (Sunnyvale, California, USA), the Prostate Cancer Foundation and the National Institute of Bioimaging and Bioengineering (R01 EB009388-01); he is also the endowed Ronald P. Lynch Professor of Urologic Oncology and Director of the LeFrak Institute of Robotic Surgery, Weill Cornell Medical College.

CHAPTER 2

Pathology of Prostate Cancer

Murali Varma[1] *and Ashish Chandra*[2]

[1]University Hospital of Wales, Cardiff, UK
[2]Guy's and St. Thomas' Hospital NHS Foundation Trust, London, UK

OVERVIEW

- Most prostate cancers are adenocarcinomas but other forms of cancer may rarely arise within the prostate

- The diagnosis of prostate cancer is based on a constellation of architectural and cytological features, almost none of which is individually diagnostic for malignancy

- Equivocal prostate biopsies are difficult to resolve due to the non-targeted nature of the biopsies and the unfeasibility of excision biopsy of the prostate gland

- Low volume cancer in prostate needle biopsies does not reliably predict minimal cancer in the prostate gland

- The Gleason grading system, which is one of the most powerful prognostic indicators of prostate cancer, is based solely on architectural features and records the most prevalent and second most prevalent grades of the tumour

---

Introduction

While prostate cancer may be suspected on clinical, biochemical and radiological grounds, in most cases, histopathology remains the only definitive diagnostic modality. Moreover, in conjunction with serum prostate specific antigen (PSA), pathology plays a pivotal role in distinguishing indolent prostate cancers that 'old men die with' from clinically significant cancers requiring radical therapy.

In this chapter, we will briefly outline the morphological features used to make a diagnosis of prostate cancer and pathological prognostic factors (with emphasis on the Gleason grading system), followed by a discussion of the role of prostate needle biopsies in contemporary management of prostate cancer.

Morphology of prostate cancer

Most prostate cancers are of prostatic glandular origin, i.e. adenocarcinoma, though occasionally other forms of cancer such as urothelial (transitional cell) carcinoma and small cell carcinoma may arise within the prostate.

The recognition of prostate cancer is made by a combination of architectural and cytological features. The architectural features that are assessed at low to medium power magnification include small, irregular shapes of glands that are closely packed together and show an infiltrative growth pattern with malignant glands extending in between normal glands. These architectural features are more difficult to appreciate in needle biopsies with a small number of atypical glands as compared to transurethral resection specimens. The most important cytological features of prostate cancer are nuclear enlargement, prominent nucleoli and the absence of a basal cell layer. Unlike the glands of prostatic adenocarcinoma that are lined by a single layer of epithelial cells, benign prostate glands that are lined by an inner layer of secretory cells and an outer layer of basal cells (Figure 2.1a). This basal cell layer may be difficult to identify on routine staining but is highlighted by immunohistochemistry for basal cell markers such as high-molecular weight cytokeratin and p63 (Figure 2.1b). However, none of these features are entirely specific for malignancy. For example, a pseudo-infiltrative pattern is often evident in benign conditions such as atrophy and the nuclear abnormalities described above may be present in benign glands adjacent to inflammation. Radiotherapy-related changes in benign glands are a particularly treacherous mimic of prostate cancer as cytological atypia in benign glandular epithelium is seen in association with a pseudo-infiltrative pattern secondary to radiation-induced atrophy. On the other hand, some variants of prostate cancer may show only minimal cytological atypia and be mistaken for benign hyperplasia or atrophy.

When several of the features of cancer and none of the features of benignity are present, the diagnosis of prostate adenocarcinoma can be made with confidence. However, in other cases, the degree of atypia may be insufficient to permit a definitive diagnosis of prostate cancer on morphologic grounds alone. These diagnostically equivocal biopsies fall into two groups.

In the first and most common situation, the changes are quantitatively insufficient to permit a definite diagnosis of cancer. These biopsies contain only a few glands lined by markedly atypical epithelial cells with all the cytological features of malignancy. However, it is recognised that larger glands with high-grade prostatic intraepithelial neoplasia (PIN) may be associated with smaller acini lined by atypical epithelial cells mimicking invasive malignancy (Figure 2.2). These 'outpouchings of PIN' are more easily identified in radical prostatectomy specimens in which the low power architecture can

---

ABC of Prostate Cancer, First Edition.
Edited by Prokar Dasgupta and Roger S. Kirby.
© 2012 Blackwell Publishing Ltd. Published 2012 by Blackwell Publishing Ltd.

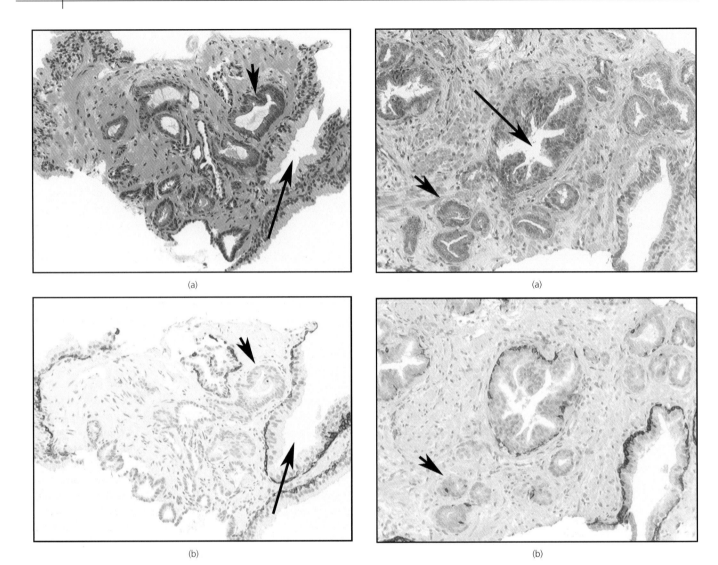

(a)

(b)

(a)

(b)

Figure 2.1 (a) Prostate needle biopsy showing small irregular malignant glands with prominent nuclear atypia (arrow heads) infiltrating between larger benign glands (arrows). (H&E stain). (b) The benign glands have an outer basal cell layer that is highlighted by immunohistochemistry using antibodies to basal cells while the malignant glands lack basal cells and are negative on immunostaining. (Immunohistochemistry: high-molecular weight cytokeratin antibody clone 34βE12).

Figure 2.2 (a) Larger gland showing features of high-grade PIN (arrow) associated with smaller glands that appear to have an infiltrative pattern suggesting prostate cancer (arrow head). (H&E).(b) Basal cell marker immunostaining shows patchy positivity in the small glands indicating that these represent outpouchings of high-grade PIN rather than cancer. (Immunohistochemistry: high-molecular weight cytokeratin antibody clone 34βE12).

be appreciated. However, in needle biopsies, the small acini may be difficult to distinguish from infiltrating cancer. Unless the small atypical glands are too numerous or too crowded to represent outpouchings, such biopsies with only a few atypical glands would be reported as 'atypical small acinar proliferation suggestive of malignancy but outpouchings of high-grade PIN cannot be excluded'.

In the other scenario, the abnormality is qualitatively insufficient for a definite diagnosis of cancer. In such cases, relatively larger foci with significant architectural distortion lack convincing cytological features of malignancy or are associated with prominent inflammation that make interpretation of the significance of cytological atypia difficult.

Prognostic factors in prostate cancer

In addition to the diagnosis of prostate cancer, histopathological examination can also provide important prognostic information to

guide patient management. The single most important pathological prognostic factor is the grade of the prostate cancer. Tumour grade refers to the degree of differentiation seen on microscopic examination, i.e. how closely the tumour resembles corresponding normal tissue. Tumours that closely resemble normal tissue are considered well differentiated or low-grade while those that are markedly different are considered poorly differentiated or high-grade.

Although there are many other systems for grading prostatic adenocarcinoma, the grading system first described by Donald Gleason in the 1960s is now almost universally employed. The Gleason system for grading prostate cancer differs from grading systems for other cancers in two important respects. Non-prostatic carcinomas are generally graded using a combination of architectural and cytological features with the highest grade recorded when a tumour shows multiple grades. In contrast, in the Gleason system, prostate cancers are graded based solely on architectural features (growth pattern and the degree of glandular differentiation) on a scale of 1 (most differentiated) to 5 (least differentiated). If multiple architectural patterns are present in a tumour, the tumour is graded using a Gleason score (also referred to as combined Gleason grade or Gleason sum), which is the sum of the primary (most prevalent) and secondary (second most prevalent) grades (e.g. Gleason score 3 + 4 = 7, when the most prevalent is 3 and the second most prevalent is 4; Gleason score 4 + 3 = 7, when the most prevalent is 4 and the second most prevalent is 3). Thus, prostate cancers are graded based on the average grade rather than worst grade. For uniformity, tumours with only a single grade are assigned a Gleason score by doubling the grade (e.g. Gleason score 3 + 3 = 6). Thus, Gleason scores could range from 2 (1+1) to 10 (5+5). However, grades 1 and 2 are practically never diagnosed on needle biopsy as they require assessment of the circumference of the tumour nodule so Gleason scores in needle biopsies generally range from 6–10. Gleason grading is applicable only to prostatic adenocarcinoma and is not used for other prostate cancers such as transitional cell carcinoma, small cell carcinoma or sarcoma. Gleason grading is also not recommended following hormonal therapy as the morphology of the tumour is altered by treatment.

Other pathological prognostic factors in prostate cancer include tumour volume and tumour stage (extent of disease within and beyond the prostate). Several biomarkers are currently being studied but none are routinely used in clinical practice.

Role of the needle biopsy in the management of prostate cancer

The role of prostatic needle biopsy has changed dramatically in recent years. In the pre-PSA era, biopsies of the prostate, generally a single transperineal 18 gauge needle biopsy, was used to confirm a clinical diagnosis of carcinoma. Now that serum PSA is used as a screening tool with a biopsy often used to sample glands that show no clinical or ultrasonographic evidence of prostate cancer, the purpose of the biopsy has become substantially different with much greater demands on the information the biopsy gives to the clinician.

Studies have found incidental, clinically unsuspected prostate cancer in 30–50% of radical cystoprostatectomies performed in men between the ages of 55 and 75 years for treatment of bladder cancer. However, only about 2% of age-matched men would be expected to die of prostate cancer. It is thus clear that a large proportion of prostate cancers in this age group are of no clinical significance. Hence, it is no longer sufficient to merely make a diagnosis of prostate cancer; pathologic features in the biopsy are used in conjunction with serum PSA levels to identify clinically significant cancers.

The most important prognostic features in the needle biopsy are the Gleason grade of the tumour and the amount of cancer in the biopsy (as determined by the number of cores involved or the extent of tumour in the cores, expressed either in mm or as a percentage involvement of core). Numerous studies have shown that the Gleason grade is a powerful predictor of outcome with Gleason scores greater than 6 being associated with a significantly

adverse outcome, as compared to lower-grade tumours. While extensive tumour in the biopsy is indicative of extensive tumour in the prostate gland and adverse outcome, the converse is not always true. Unlike breast cancer where the abnormality in the breast is identified clinically by palpation or radiologically by mammogram followed by targeted biopsy of the lesion, most early prostate cancers cannot be accurately localised by clinical or radiological examination. In the latter situation, the identified abnormality in the blood (raised serum PSA) is followed by non-targeted systematic sampling of the prostate gland which may result in a 'tip of the iceberg' phenomenon. Hence, minimal tumour in prostate biopsies may be associated with extensive tumour in the prostate gland and it is critically important that the pathologist diligently screens prostate biopsies to identify even tiny foci of cancer.

The non-targeted nature of prostate biopsies also results in a significant false negative rate: about 25% with traditional six core sextant biopsies. The presence of high-grade prostatic intraepithelial neoplasia (PIN), a precursor lesion for most prostate cancers (analogous to DCIS of the breast), in an otherwise negative prostate biopsy, has been used to identify a subset of patients for repeat needle biopsy because they are at a higher risk of having co-existing cancer that has been missed at the first biopsy. The frequency of missed cancer is much lower in contemporary practice with at least eight cores taken from the prostate gland so repeat biopsies may not be warranted if isolated high-grade PIN is found following use of such extended biopsy protocols.

Another major problem with prostatic needle biopsy relates to the difficulty in resolving cases in which the diagnosis is uncertain. A biopsy diagnosis of 'suspicious but not diagnostic for malignancy' in other organs such as the breast and the lung can be resolved by targeted repeat biopsy or excision of the abnormality for definitive histological examination. In contrast, prostate biopsies are non-targeted, hence a negative re-biopsy following a diagnosis of 'suspicious for adenocarcinoma' does not exclude malignancy as the second biopsy may be a false negative. Moreover, excision biopsy is not a feasible alternative for resolving equivocal prostate biopsies as the suspect focus cannot be accurately localised. Hence, the pathologist must make every effort to avoid equivocal prostate needle biopsy reports by taking extreme care with the technical aspects of processing needle cores and in the interpretation of the biopsies.

Further reading

Epstein JI. An update on the Gleason grading system. *J Urology* 2010;**183**: 433–40.

Harnden P, Berney D, Shelley M. *Prostate cancer dataset*, The Royal College of Pathologists. http://www.rcpath.org/resources/pdf/g084dataset prostaticcarcinomaoct09.pdf.

Varma M, Griffiths DFR. Equivocal prostate needle biopsies. In Bowsher W, Carter A. (eds) *Challenges in prostate cancer*. Oxford: Blackwell, 76–84, 2006.

Varma M, Lee MW, Tamboli P, Zarbo RJ, Jimenez R, Salles PG et al. Morphologic criteria for the diagnosis of prostatic adenocarcinoma in needle biopsy specimens. *Arch Pathol Lab Med* 2002;**126**:554–61.

CHAPTER 3

Biology of Prostate Cancer

R. William G. Watson[1] *and John M. Fitzpatrick*[2]

[1]UCD School of Medicine and Medical Science, Conway Institute of Biomolecular and Biomedical Research, University College Dublin, Dublin, Ireland
[2]UCD School of Medicine and Medical Science, Mater Misericordiae University Hospital, University College Dublin, Dublin, Ireland

OVERVIEW

- Prostate cancer is a heterogeneous disease
- Development and progression of disease are influenced by genetic and environmental factors
- Combinations of germline mutations are most likely to contribute to cancer development
- Gene fusions represent important rearrangements which may help to explain somatic changes in prostate cancer
- Environmental changes influenced by ageing may represent important factors contributing to the biology of prostate cancer

Introduction

Knowledge of the molecular and cellular mechanisms of prostate cancer will inform men's risk of disease and progression and direct the development of diagnostic and therapeutic interventions. As in most cancers, it is presumed that prostate cancer develops from a single cell that undergoes genetic changes influenced by the environment, which in turn affects the regulation of the cell resulting in a survival advantage, genetic instability and eventually tumourogenesis (Figure 3.1). This chapter divides the mechanisms of prostate cancer into genetic (inherited, somatic and epigenetic changes) and physiological factors (ageing, tissue remodelling, chronic inflammation and hypoxia) which may contribute to the heterogenic nature of the disease.

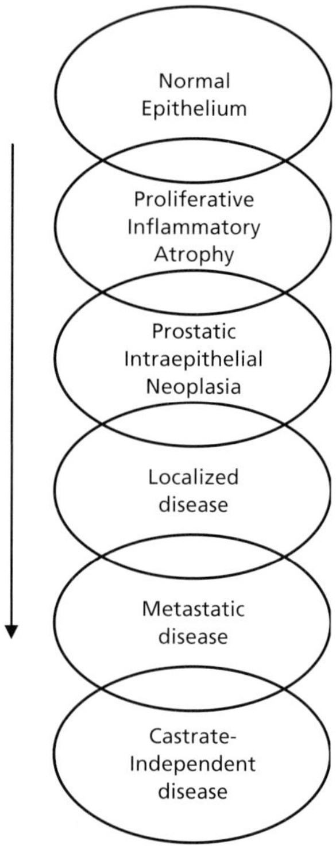

Figure 3.1 Proposed progression of prostate cancer.

Genetic factors

Germline mutations

Prostate cancer has been shown to cluster in families with 5–10% associated with a substantial inherited component. Significant advances have been made in the past 5–10 years in the area of susceptibility genes and gene fusions (Table 3.1). Similar to breast cancer, high-risk prostate cancer is associated with a germline mutation in BRCA2 with a five times greater risk of prostate cancer and the development of more aggressive disease. However, BRCA2 mutations only account for 2% of disease onset, indicating that other susceptibility loci exit. There is now evidence to suggest that prostate cancer inheritance is complex with numerous low penetrance genes associated with its development. Initially ELAC2, MSR1 and RNASEL were identified as candidate genes. More recent evidence has identified an additional 10 susceptibility loci and highlighted candidate genes including MSMB, KLK3 and LMTK2. Polymorphic variants have also been identified which could contribute to sporadic cases of prostate cancer. These include single nucleotide polymorphisms (SNPs) in genes involved in the action of androgens, which is centrally involved in regulating growth, differentiation and survival of prostate epithelial cells. These genes include the androgen-receptor, CYP17, which encodes cytochrome P-450c17α (an enzyme that catalyzes key reactions in sex-steroid biosynthesis) and the steroid 5-α-reductase type II

ABC of Prostate Cancer, First Edition.
Edited by Prokar Dasgupta and Roger S. Kirby.

Table 3.1 Gene involved in prostate cancer development.

Observation	Gene
Higher levels in cancer than in normal prostate	Telomerase
	E2F4
	Activated MAPK
	DD3 PCA3
	PIM1
	Hepsin
	AMACR
Lower levels in cancer than in normal prostate	PTEN
	E-cadherin
	IGFBP-3
	GSTP1
Higher levels in metastases than in primary tumour	c-met
	Cyclin E1
	MTA-1
	EZH2
Higher levels in castrate independent than in androgen dependent	bcl-2
	p21
	fibronectin
	IGFBP-2
	Insulin receptor
Lower levels in castrate independent than in androgen dependent	BTG-1
	Oncostatin-M

Source: Adapted from Foley et al Endocrine-related cancer 11: 477–488, 2004. © Society for Endocrinology (2004). Reproduced by permission.

Table 3.2 Somatic events in prostate cancer.

Gene	Change observed	Function
ETS family	Translocation downstream of AR-regulated genes	Transcription factors that regulate differentiation and growth
GSTP1	Methylation of promoter	Presents oxidation stress
PTEN	Loss	Regulation of cellular metabolism and proliferation
NKX3.1	Loss/inactivation	Regulation of epithelial growth and differentiation
c-myc	Gene amplification	Regulation of cell proliferation, autophagy and apoptosis
Rb	Loss (LOH, mutation)	Regulation of cell cycle
P53	Loss (LOH, mutation)	Detection of damaged DNA, regulation of cell cycle and apoptosis
AR	Amplification, mutation	Regulation of cell differentiation and proliferation

Source: Adapted from Febbo PG. Genomic approaches to outcome prediction in prostate cancer. *Cancer* 2009;**111**(13Suppl):3046–57. Reproduced by permission from Wiley.

which is the predominant isozyme that converts testosterone to the more potent dihydrotestosterone. Mutations in these genes have been linked to increased risk of prostate cancer development. A novel susceptibility locus has also been identified on chromosome 22, and polymorphisms on chromosomes 8 and 17 are linked to disease development with a combination of five SNPs increasing an individual's risk by fivefold.

Somatic defects

Where germline mutations contribute to genetic changes associated with prostate cancer development, there is also an accumulation of other genetic changes, including gene deletions, gene amplifications, chromosomal rearrangements and epigenetic changes (DNA methylation), that occur over time (Table 3.2). Advances in high throughput technology have helped to increase our understanding and research findings in this area, however, due to the heterogenecity of prostate tumours, results often vary between studies. The most common chromosomal abnormalities are gains at 7p, 7q, 8q, and Xq and losses at 8p, 10q, 13q and 16q. The stage of the disease increases with increasing genetic alterations, suggesting an accumulation of genetic abnormalities. Loss of 8p is seen in high grade PIN (precursor lesion to prostate cancer).

Epigenetic changes in prostate cancer include DNA methylation alterations and histone modifications and both can lead to chromosomal instability and the silencing of genes. The ability to reverse epigenetic changes to reactivate silent genes could be a potential therapeutic strategy in the future. One of the earliest epigenetic changes is the hypermethylation of GSTP1, which encodes for glutathione S-transferase which protects against toxic metabolites

preventing genome damage. Loss of GSTP1 has been shown in 90% of prostate cancer cases. NKX3.1 encodes a prostate-specific homeobox gene which has been shown to be involved in normal prostate development and binds DNA, repressing expression of the PSA gene. Loss of its expression by gene deletions or rearrangements occurs early in prostate cancer development and in about 90% of cases. Loss of PTEN expression is also associated with prostate cancer development. PTEN represents a centrally important regulator of AKT activation which is a central regulator of growth, differentiation and survival and a key signalling pathway in prostate cancer development and progression. Additional stimulation of cancer cell proliferation can occur by reduced expression of p27, a cyclin-dependent kinase inhibitor encoded by the CDKN1B gene which is common in localised and metastatic prostate cancer. This loss of p27 may occur by either AKT activation or somatic loss of 12p12-13 which encompasses CDKN1B. Increased cell number is also regulated by apoptosis and rates of apoptosis have been shown to be altered during initiation, progression and metastasis of prostate cancer. Androgen withdrawal results in the induction of apoptosis and the over-expression of different survival proteins, including Bcl-2 and inhibitors of the apoptosis family of proteins. It also prevents this cell death and is associated with castrate-independent disease. One fundamental new concept that has emerged from castrate-resistant disease is the tumour's ability to synthesise its own androgen. This self-sufficiency in the central growth and survival factor of the prostate allows the cell to survive traditional androgen depletion strategies.

Other up-regulated genes include MYC, an oncogene which is amplified in prostate cancer and associated with the development of PIN-like lesions, prostate carcinoma as well as poor prognosis.

The ETS genes have also been associated with the development of prostate cancer. They co-operate with other transcription factors to regulate proliferation, differentiation, angiogenesis, oncogenic transformation and apoptosis. Normally suppressed in prostate epithelial cells, they have been shown to be up-regulated through fusion with the androgen-responsive gene TMPRSS2, as a result of rearrangements. The TMPRSS2:ERG gene fusion is observed in the majority of prostate cancer cases. Seventeen different types of TMPRSS2:ERG fusion transcripts have been identified.

Although we know much about the genetics of prostate cancer there is no clear genetic model.

Environmental factors

There are also physiological factors that contribute to the development of prostate cancer such as ageing, tissue remodelling, inflammation and hypoxia.

Ageing

One of the most significant risk factors for the development of prostate cancer is age. Ageing has been associated with progressive changes of physiological functions leading to changes in tissue hypoxia, suppression of the immune system ('immunosenescence'), alterations in hormone levels and in DNA repair mechanisms. Ageing is also associated with DNA mutations and alterations in repair mechanisms which increase the risk of cancer. Reactive oxygen species and lack of repair contribute to mitochondrial DNA damage which has been shown to exist in prostate cancer.

Tissue remodelling

The ageing prostate undergoes structural changes known as remodelling which leads to alterations in gene expression affecting cellular processes such as apoptosis, proliferation and steroid signalling. These alterations play an important role in carcinogenesis, with a modified stroma (reactive stroma) leading to a more favourable microenvironment for tumour growth. Tissue remodelling, which occurs as a result of hormonal alterations and diet, is thought to result in hypoxia which may then contribute to the development of early prostate cancer.

The transforming growth factor (TGFβ) is thought to play a major role in the development of a reactive stroma and the initiation of prostate cancer. It is secreted from the hypertrophic basal cell layer. TGFβ is a cytokine involved in cell proliferation and differentiation and its inhibition is lost in the progression of prostate cancer. TGFβ further enhances stroma remodelling through increased expression of proteolytic matrix metalloproteinases and causes differentiation of smooth muscle cells and stromal fibroblasts into myofibroblasts. The changes in growth factor then alter epithelial/stromal cell interactions and lead to inappropriate growth of prostate epithelial cells. Cell proliferation results in an imbalance between the oxygen supply and the oxygen demand of proliferating cells. Hypoxia inducible factor 1alpha (HIF−1α) up-regulates hypoxia-responsive genes such as fibroblast growth factor-2 and factor-7 (FGF-2 and FGF-7), VEGF and GLUT-1. The altered expression of cell secretions leads to the clogging of ducts and an inflammatory response which may increase levels of hypoxia.

Chronic inflammation

Chronic inflammation has been linked to cancer in several disease models; it causes cell and genome damage, promoting cellular turnover and creating a tissue micro-environment that can enhance cell replication, angiogenesis and tissue repair. It is found frequently in radical prostatectomy and biopsy specimens. Studies have shown common molecular pathways between inflammation and cancer development in the prostate.

Chronic inflammation occurs in the prostate secondary to both infectious and noxious agents and is associated with atypical hyperplasia of the prostate epithelium with dysplastic changes. Inflammation also leads to the production of free radicals and COX-2 activity through infiltrating macrophages and neutrophils. GSTP1, which usually protects the cell from genomic damage, is methylated (as discussed above) and cannot prevent this DNA damage.

Proliferative inflammatory atrophy (PIA), which shares some molecular traits with prostate intraepithelial neoplasia and prostate cancer, has been characterised as areas of atrophy with high numbers of inflammatory cells. PIA occurs as a result of repeated injury and is most commonly found in the peripheral zone where the majority of cancer cells are found. Repeated insults lead to additional changes such as loss of tumour suppressor gene PTEN. This may lead to activation of the AKT pathway and subsequent NFKB and HIF activation.

Conclusion

Prostate cancer is a complex heterogeneous disease with multiple contributing factors which have complicated our understanding of its development and progression.

Further reading

Elo J, Visakorpi T. Molecular genetics of prostate cancer. *Ann Med* 2001; **33**:130–41.

Febbo PG. Genomic approaches to outcome prediction in prostate cancer. *Cancer* 2009;**115** (13 Suppl):3046–57.

Foley F, Hollywood D, LawlerM. Molecular pathology of prostate cancer: The key to identifying new biomarkers of disease. *Endocrine-related cancer*. 2004;**11**:477–88.

Mackinnon AC, Yan BC, Joseph LJ, Al-Ahmadie HA. Molecular biology underlying the clinical heterogeneity of prostate cancer: An update. *Arch Pathol Lab Med* 2009;**133**:1033–40.

Nelson WG, DeMarzo AM, Isaacs WB. Prostate cancer. *N Eng J Med* 2003;**349**:366–81.

CHAPTER 4

Prostate Cancer Diagnosis

Robin Weston[1,2,3], Anthony J. Costello[1,2] and Declan G. Murphy[2,4]

[1]Department of Urology, The Royal Melbourne Hospital, Melbourne, VIC, Australia
[2]Department of Urology, The Peter MacCallum Cancer Centre, Melbourne, VIC, Australia
[3]The Australian Prostate Cancer Research Centre, Epworth Richmond Hospital, Melbourne, VIC, Australia
[4]University of Melbourne, Melbourne, VIC, Australia

OVERVIEW

- Clinical presentation of prostate cancer
- Diagnostic role and limitations of PSA and DRE
- Prostate biopsy techniques
- Limited role of imaging in the diagnosis
- PCA-3 testing

Table 4.1 Presenting symptoms for advanced prostate cancer.

Locally advanced	Metastatic
Obstructive LUTS	Bone pain
Haematuria	Pathological fracture
Haematospermia	Anaemia
Pain (penile, perineal)	Lower limb/inguinal oedema
Obstructive uropathy	Hypercalcaemia
Erectile dysfunction	

Presentation

Due to stage migration caused by increased use of the prostate cancer antigen (PSA) testing, the majority of men diagnosed with prostate cancer now present with the localised disease. Early prostate cancer (PC) is invariably asymptomatic and is usually identified in patients who are found to have an elevated serum prostate-specific antigen and/or an abnormal digital rectal examination (DRE). Although the use of PSA testing and DRE in asymptomatic men is currently contentious, this remains the most reliable way of diagnosing men with early prostate cancer who can then choose between a range of curative interventions or a period of active surveillance.

Lower urinary tract symptoms (LUTS) are common in men over the age of 50 years and are usually secondary to benign prostatic hyperplasia, however, prostate cancer can also cause these symptoms and as both diseases often co-exist, it is important that PC is ruled out. Advanced prostate cancer can present with local or distant symptoms, as outlined in Table 4.1. The peripheral location of most cancers can also be the reason why even advanced prostate cancer may cause little or no lower urinary tract symptoms.

Obstructive uropathy can be either the result of bladder outflow obstruction or bilateral ureteric infiltration at the level of the trigone, and the latter must be suspected if renal function does not improve following catheter drainage of the bladder. Erectile dysfunction (ED) is another symptom which is relatively common in the age group of men at risk of prostate cancer and it is probably more likely to be incidental, however, as noted above, PC often co-exists with LUTS and ED, therefore, it is important to rule

out significant underlying PC. A DRE should be performed, and patients should be counselled about the merits of a PSA test in their particular circumstances.

Bone is the most common site for metastatic PC with a predilection for the axial skeleton, particularly the lower back, pelvis and hips. Although less common, symptomatic bone metastases are still the presenting symptom of advanced prostate cancer for men who have not previously had a PSA test and/or DRE. In the case of bone metastasis, plain X-rays may show sclerotic deposits, and an isotope bone scan may be helpful to confirm the presence of metastasis. This diagnosis must be considered particularly in men over the age of 70 presenting with axial bone pain.

First step: serum PSA and digital rectal examination

PSA is an enzyme in the form of a 237 amino acid glycoprotein produced primarily by cells lining the acini and ducts of the prostate gland. Its main biological function is the dissolution of the gel-forming proteins in the freshly ejaculated semen. PSA is also present in normal male serum in small quantities, and is often elevated in prostate cancer. It is, however, not specific to prostate cancer and can be elevated by other conditions such as benign prostate hyperplasia, urinary tract infection, inflammation and trauma (such as catheterisation). Hence, PSA levels tend to increase as men age, regardless of whether or not they have underlying prostate cancer. Approximately 25% of patients with a level of 4–10 ng/ml will be identified as having prostate cancer on biopsy. More recently, clinicians have adopted a more refined approach to PSA testing in an attempt to improve its sensitivity and specificity utilising age-adjusted levels (Table 4.2), PSA isoforms, PSA density and PSA velocity. Early PSA testing in men in their forties has been advocated by some to predict the future risk of developing cancer.

Table 4.2 Age-specific reference ranges for serum PSA.

Age range	PSA reference range
40–49 yr	0–2.5 ng/mL
50–59 yr	0–3.5 ng/mL
60–69 yr	0–4.5 ng/mL
70–79 yr	0–6.5 ng/mL

Source: Richardson, T.D. and Oesterling, J.E.: Age-specific reference ranges for serum prostatespecific antigen. *Urol Clin North Am*, 1997;**24**:339.

The value of a digital rectal examination (DRE)

A DRE can detect palpable prostate cancer even in the early disease stage as it generally occurs on the periphery of the gland. In localised disease where the cancer is confined to the prostate, the clinician may palpate a firm nodule within the prostate. Once the gland feels very abnormal with an irregular outline or distorted anatomy, it often suggests that the disease is locally advanced. As with any examination skill, the clinician must perform many examinations to appreciate normal prostatic variation before being able to confidently identify an abnormal or suspicious gland. The importance of performing a digital rectal examination in the diagnosis of PC cannot be over-emphasised and should not be omitted because of the false assumption that PSA testing or imaging is superior. First, patients with a normal PSA may harbour a prostate cancer either in the case of an early small volume but palpable disease or in advanced poorly differentiated non-PSA-secreting prostate cancer, both of which could easily be missed without a DRE. Furthermore, trans-rectal ultra-sonography or magnetic resonance imaging is generally not used for detecting prostate cancer and is reserved for localising biopsies or staging, once the diagnosis has been confirmed. DRE should be considered an essential adjunct to PSA testing.

Confirmation of the diagnosis – a prostate biopsy

If the clinician has any clinical or biochemical suspicion of prostate cancer, the diagnosis can be confirmed by taking a biopsy. This is most commonly performed by following the trans-rectal ultrasound-guided approach (TRUS) using a tru-cut needle. The procedure is usually performed in the clinic under local anaesthetic with or without sedation (see Figure 4.1). A general anaesthetic is occasionally required. A sextant biopsy (i.e. six cores) were traditionally taken, however, this was associated with around a 30% false negative rate and an extended biopsy scheme utilising a 12-core biopsy strategy is now recommended.

The value of a prostate biopsy is much more than just establishing the presence or not of malignancy. As clinicians have become aware of the degree of over-diagnosis and over-treatment which has accompanied the increased use of PSA testing, considerable effort has been made to identify men at low risk of disease progression and therefore who are suitable for surveillance rather than intervention. Therefore, prostate biopsies are used to establish the volume, grade and multifocal nature of the tumour so patients and clinicians can better predict their likely outcome.

The risks and complications of prostate biopsy include haematuria, haematospermia, urinary retention, perineal discomfort,

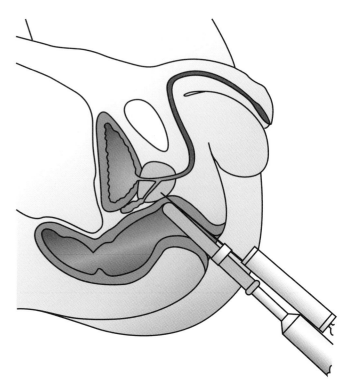

Figure 4.1 Trans-rectal ultrasound-guided biopsy of the prostate.

Table 4.3 Complications of trans-rectal prostate biopsy.

Complication	Frequency (%)	Comment
Haematuria	23–63	0.7% clot retention
Haematospermia	10–50	Up to 6 weeks
Rectal bleeding	2–21	Usually minor
Infection	2.5–10	2% requiring hospitalisation
Urinary retention	0.4	
Vasovagal episode	1.4–5.3	
Pain		Local anaesthetic and/or sedation mandatory

Source: Campbell-Walsh Urology, 2007, with permission from Elsevier.

urinary tract infection and septicaemia (see Table 4.3). The use of antibiotic prophylaxis has reduced infection rates from 25% to less than 10%. Typical antibiotic prophylactic schemes would include a one-off dose of an aminoglycoside or a short course of fluroquinolone, or a combination of both. Infection post biopsy is therefore now relatively uncommon but occasionally serious with about 2% of patients requiring hospitalization for severe infection.

The role of repeat biopsy

In patients who have a persistent clinical suspicion of prostate cancer, despite previous negative prostate biopsies, some clinicians will employ a saturation biopsy technique where typically 24–32 prostate cores are taken.

More recently, a trans-perineal template-guided biopsy has been employed with endorectal ultra-sound guidance (Figure 4.2). This technique can allow more accurate sampling of the entire

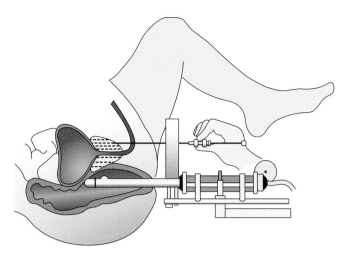

Figure 4.2 Trans-perineal template biopsy of the prostate.

prostate and may achieve better access to apical and transitional zone tissue, thereby increasing cancer detection rates. The traditional method of finger guided tru-cut trans-rectal biopsy is now utilised less frequently although can still be useful to sample a palpable nodule.

Prostate cancer diagnosed at transurethral resection of the prostate (TURP)

Occasionally, the histological diagnosis of prostate cancer is made when analysing the resected tissue from a transurethral resection of the prostate(TURP). The urologist may have suspicions of prostate cancer when undertaking the procedure although the pathological report may sometimes be the first indication of any underlying problem. As a TURP usually resects the transition zone, and prostate cancer arises from the peripheral zone, further biopsies may still be required to fully stage the diagnosis.

The main risk factor for PC is age, being relatively rare below the age of 40 and rising rapidly over the age of 70. Other risk factors include: family history, with the risk doubling with one first degree relative having PC; ethnicity, highest among African-Americans and lowest among East Asians, and nationality, North Americans and Europeans have a higher incidence than Asians and Latin Americans. Numerous dietary factors including fat intake, calcium, lycopene (found in cooked tomatoes) and trace elements such as selenium have been implicated with either increasing or reducing the risk of prostate cancer, although all these studies have significant confounding factors.

Prostate cancer can be incidentally found following histological examination of TURP chips, however, since the widespread introduction of PSA testing, this has become less common.

The use of imaging for diagnosis of prostate cancer

There is no place for diagnostic imaging in the routine diagnosis of prostate cancer. Imaging modalities such as MRI may be useful for staging cancer which has already been diagnosed (and may be used to guide prostate biopsies in certain circumstances), and trans-rectal ultrasound is essential to systematically guide biopsies, but otherwise imaging is not used as a primary diagnostic tool. One exception is the use of an isotope bone scan and/or plain X-rays to confirm the presence of metastatic disease in patients presenting with bone-related symptoms and a very high PSA. In these circumstances, clinical suspicion and a positive bone scan are sufficient to make the diagnosis without a biopsy.

Novel approaches to diagnosis of prostate cancer

A novel test, which is currently becoming more widespread in the detection of prostate cancer, is based on the PCA-3 gene, discovered in the 1990s. PCA-3 is highly expressed in prostate cancer and found in very low levels in benign prostatic tissue. The Progensa™ PCA-3 test (manufactured by Gen-Probe, San Diego, CA, USA) is used to analyze urine samples collected after the DRE. In fact, it is a dual assay which quantifies both PCA-3 and PSA mRNA to produce a ratio which can then be used to calculate PC risk. The test appears to be more cancer-specific than serum PSA and, unlike PSA, is not known to be influenced by BPH or other factors such as trauma, inflammation or age.

Reference

Campbell Walsh (2007) *Urology.* 9th edn. Edited by AJ Wein, LR Kavoussi, AC Novick, AW Partin, CA Peters. New York: Elsevier.

Further reading

Richardson, T.D. and Oesterling, J.E. Age-specific reference ranges for serum prostatespecific antigen. *Urol Clin North Am*, 1997;**24**:339.
EAU Guidelines on Prostate Cancer (www.uroweb.org).

CHAPTER 5

Imaging of Prostate Cancer

James Halls and Uday Patel

Department of Radiology, St George's Healthcare NHS Trust, London, UK

OVERVIEW

- The role of imaging in prostate cancer diagnosis and staging in standard clinical practice
- The differing roles of the various imaging modalities: plain imaging, trans-rectal ultrasound (TRUS), CT, MRI and isotope bone scans and how they are integrated into clinical practice
- For each of the imaging modalities, an understanding of the typical appearances of prostate cancer and potential difficulties with their use
- Potential future imaging modalities

Introduction

Although prostate cancer is occasionally an incidental finding during radiological investigations for other purposes, the main focus of prostate cancer imaging is to both aid in the diagnosis and provide accurate staging of both local and advanced disease. Accurate staging is essential for treatment planning. For example, advanced local disease would be inappropriately treated with radical prostatectomy, with unnecessary potential patient morbidity while burdening healthcare resources.

In standard practice, trans-rectal ultrasound (TRUS) provides only limited diagnostic and staging information but is essential for guiding prostatic biopsy. MRI and bone scans are used for cancer staging, while CT is reserved for advanced/metastatic disease. Table 5.1 presents a summary of the features of each kind of imaging used in prostate cancer detection.

Plain imaging

The prostate is the commonest primary site for sclerotic bone metastases in men and the identification of such lesions, which may be an incidental finding in those with skeletal pain, may be the prompt for further assessment with digital rectal examination (DRE) and/or measurement of the prostate specific antigen

Table 5.1 Summary of types of imaging.

Type	Features
Plain imaging	Bone metastases typically sclerotic
	Destructive metastases in long bones carry a risk of pathological fracture
TRUS	Typically requested after abnormal DRE or elevated PSA measurement
	Prostate cancer hypoechoic and located in peripheral zone
	Overall sensitivity too low to use as a sole diagnostic tool
	Main role is to guide systematic prostatic biopsies
MRI	Main imaging modality to assess local disease extent and staging
	Endorectal MRI improves resolution but is uncomfortable and not standard practise
	Cancer foci appear as low signal lesions within background high signal of peripheral zone
	Allows identification of extracapsular spread, seminal vesicle involvement and pelvic lymph node staging
	Delay of 4–8 weeks following biopsy advised to avoid confusion from post-biopsy haemorrhage
CT	Poor contrast resolution limits role in assessing local disease extent
	Used for assessment of organ and lymph node metastases
Bone scan	Modality of choice for identification of bone metastases
	Metastases manifest as foci of increased tracer uptake, appearing 'hot' relative to background skeleton
	Typically reserved for 'high-risk' patients
	Can occasionally miss small metastatic foci (for which MRI is better)

(PSA) level. Widespread sclerotic lesions in an elderly male patient should be regarded as likely metastatic prostate cancer until proven otherwise. The presence of destructive lesions within long bones is associated with a risk of pathological fracture. With the advent of more modern imaging modalities, plain imaging has only a limited role in the management of prostate cancer.

Trans-rectal ultrasound (TRUS)

The anatomical position of the prostate immediately anterior to the rectum lends itself well to trans-rectal ultrasound with a high-frequency (5–7.5 MHz) probe. Since its introduction in 1971, TRUS has become the commonest imaging modality of the prostate,

---

ABC of Prostate Cancer, First Edition.
Edited by Prokar Dasgupta and Roger S. Kirby.
© 2012 Blackwell Publishing Ltd. Published 2012 by Blackwell Publishing Ltd.

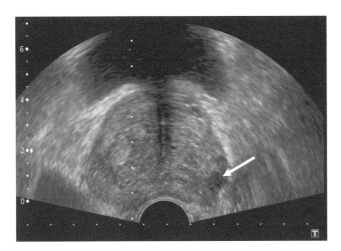

Figure 5.1 Transverse section TRUS image of a prostate. Note the small rounded hypoechoic (dark) focus within the left periphery of the gland (white arrow). Targeted biopsy proved carcinoma of the prostate.

typically requested after an abnormal DRE or elevated PSA measurement. Prostate cancer is typically hypoechoic (dark) and located in the peripheral zone (see Figure 5.1). Unfortunately, most cancers are either isoechoic (i.e. the same shade of grey) as the surrounding tissue or of non-specific appearance, indistinguishable from background benign prostate hyperplasia. Diagnostic specificity is especially poor in the central gland, within the heterogeneous-appearing transition zone.

Extracapsular extension (stage T3a disease) is also poorly visualised but suggested by local capsular bulging or irregularity. Extension into the seminal vesicles (stage T3b disease) is suggested by solid hypoechoic lesions within the cystic (anechoic – very dark) vesicles. Like all tumours, prostate cancer has associated neovascularisation and the additional use of Doppler ultrasound (which identifies blood flow) can improve diagnostic specificity.

Despite this, the overall sensitivity of TRUS in cancer identification is too low to allow its use as a sole diagnostic tool. As a consequence, its main role is in guiding trans-rectal biopsy. As most cancers are sonographically invisible, prostate biopsy is a sampling technique and multiple, systematic biopsies of the entire gland are necessary. The number of cores necessary for adequate sampling has increased over the years, a consequence of the downward stage migration of prostate cancer. Current recommendations are for at least 10–12 cores targeted onto the peripheral zone, but some centres use more. At its most extreme, 'saturation biopsies' are undertaken where 24 or more cores are taken. Naturally this improved sampling results in higher accuracy but this comes at the expense of diagnosing small volume, possibly insignificant, cancers and extra morbidity. Other applications for TRUS in prostate cancer management include measurement of prostatic volume (which allows calculation of PSA density) and guidance for brachytherapy seed implantation.

Computed tomography (CT)

The role of CT in assessing local prostate cancer extent is limited by its poor contrast resolution, with the gland being indistinguishable from the adjacent bladder base and seminal vesicles. Its role is reserved for staging of advanced disease and typically for assessment of organ and lymph node metastases. As a guide, in asymptomatic patients with a PSA <20 ng/ml, CT is generally not required due to the low (<1%) probability of a positive study. Similarly, in cases of localised disease, CT detects lymphadenopathy in <1%, the figure increasing to almost 20% with locally advanced disease. Lymphadenopathy is demonstrated in 1% of patients with a Gleason score of less than or equal to 7, increasing to 12.5% with a score of 8 or higher. Other uses include demonstration of sclerotic bone metastases or evaluation of suspicious areas identified on radioisotope bone scans.

Magnetic resonance imaging (MRI)

Unlike CT, MRI is vastly superior for soft tissue resolution and is the best imaging modality for local disease assessment and staging. Endorectal MRI has better spatial resolution but is an uncomfortable examination and standard pelvic (external) coils are the preferred method in most centres. On T1-weighted studies, the gland is of uniformly low/mid -signal intensity and neither the normal prostate zonal anatomy or tumours are seen. T2-weighted images are the sequence of choice for both appreciation of zonal anatomy and cancer detection. Prostate cancer appears as round or ill-defined foci of low signal intensity (dark), highlighted against the normally high signal (bright) peripheral zone (PZ), where the majority of cancers arise (see Figure 5.2). Evaluation of the central gland is a problem on MRI too, as the lower signal intensity masks any inner gland tumours and the heterogenous appearance of the TZ further reduces the diagnostic specificity.

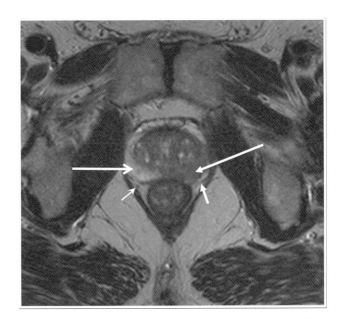

Figure 5.2 Axial T2-weighted MRI image of prostate cancer. Note the focal area of abnormal low signal (dark) change within the left peripheral zone posterolaterally (long closed arrow). Compare with the normal high signal (white) peripheral zone of the right aspect of the gland (long open arrow). There is no evidence of bulging/breach of the adjacent low signal thin prostatic capsule (short closed arrow) to suggest extracapsular extension. The neurovascular bundles run in the 7 o'clock position (arrowhead).

The neurovascular bundles run adjacent to the thin stripe of the prostatic capsule. Features of extra-capsular spread include local capsular bulging and asymmetry of the neurovascular bundles. This is an important finding as the upstaging impacts on treatment choice. The overall accuracy of MRI in identifying capsular penetration is mixed with figures quoted between 33–82%. The maximum sensitivity for detecting extracapsular spread has been quoted at 64%. Seminal vesicle invasion especially influences the treatment choices. These paired high signal structures appear as bunch-of-grape-like structures lying posterior to the base of the bladder. Invasion is suggested by abnormal low signal replacing the normal high signal. MRI evaluation of disease stage is rarely straightforward. In repeated studies, the overall, accuracy is in the 70–80% range, although some specialised centres do report much better figures. Many factors conspire to limit accuracy. One commonly encountered problem is post-biopsy haemorrhage. Similar to cancer, this appears as low signal foci on T2-weighted imaging, although, in contrast to cancer, it is generally of high signal on T1 images. To avoid diagnostic uncertainty, most practitioners advise a delay of 4–8 weeks following biopsy prior to MRI.

In addition to local staging, MRI has other uses such as pelvic lymph node staging, confirmation of bone metastases (for example, if equivocal on isotope bone scans) and identification of associated problems such as potentially catastrophic spinal cord compression.

Radionuclide bone scintigraphy (bone scan)

Bone deposits are the commonest manifestation of prostate cancer metastases and the risk rises with increasing PSA level and Gleason grade. They have a predilection for the axial skeleton, such as the pelvis, vertebrae and ribs. A radioisotope bone scan is the modality of choice for their detection. A study involves an intravenous injection of 99mTc (the radioisotope which emits gamma rays) linked to a phosphonate (which allows skeletal uptake). Prostate cancer metastases are osteoblastic and associated with increased tracer uptake, appearing 'hot' relative to the background skeleton (Figure 5.3). The technique has a very high sensitivity. In a patient with a significantly elevated PSA, multiple areas of increased uptake within the axial skeleton are virtually diagnostic for metastatic disease. Interpretation difficulty occurs with other causes of increased bone turnover, such as spinal degenerative disease or rib fractures. Correlation with plain films or MRI imaging will help resolve these difficult cases.

The potential for bone metastases rises with increasing PSA levels. Abuzallouf et al. (2004) performed a meta-analysis and reported that a PSA <10 ng/ml carries a 2.3% chance of a bone scan being positive. Levels of 10–20 and 20–50 have a risk of 5.3% and 16.2% respectively. If disease is confined to the prostate, the chance of bone metastases is around 6%, increasing to nearly 50% with locally advanced disease. A Gleason score of less than or equal to 7 is associated with a 5.6% chance of bone metastases, which increases to almost 30% with a score of 8 or above. As such, a bone scan should be considered if the PSA is above 20, locally advanced disease or a Gleason score is >8.

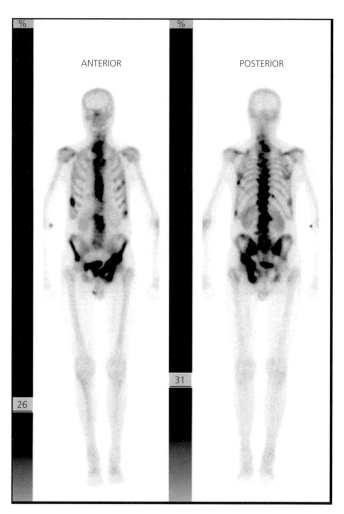

Figure 5.3 Multiple prostatic bone metastases on isotope bone scan. Note the multiple foci of abnormal uptake scattered throughout the ribs, vertebrae and pelvis. The PSA at the time of the study was greater than 1200.

Potential or future imaging modalities

This final section will cover potential new imaging modalities that may improve specificity or sensitivity of prostate cancer detection. It is worth stressing that these modalities are not routinely available and many remain experimental at best.

TRUS with microbubble enhancement is a strategy to better demonstrate cancer-associated neo-vascularity. An intravascular sonographically visible agent is injected intravenously while the prostate is assessed in real time with either colour or power Doppler imaging. Foci of increased vascularity can be specifically targeted for biopsy. This may pick up cancer foci that might otherwise be missed due to sampling error with the systematic approach. Elastography is another technique under investigation. Simplistically, it is the ultrasound equivalent of the DRE, being sensitive to areas of reduced tissue elasticity.

MRI spectroscopy adds metabolic information to a standard MRI image. It works on the principle that prostate cancers secrete smaller or larger amounts of certain metabolites (principally citrate, choline and creatine) than normal prostatic tissue. The aim is to demonstrate abnormal metabolite levels in keeping with cancer.

It has been suggested that the technique could aid in PZ cancer detection and a possible relationship between Gleason grade and magnitude of the chemical ratio abnormality proposed. However, it requires an exacting technique that is not easily reproducible and has not translated into everyday practice.

Dynamic MRI also works on the principle of neo-vascularity and involves the rapid injection of low-molecular weight contrast agent with subsequent fast MRI imaging of the prostate every 20–30 seconds. Cancers are reported to show early enhancement and early contrast washout. This may be further exaggerated with higher grade cancers. Diffusion-weighted MRI (DWI) utilises the principle of Brownian motion of water molecules within tissues. In general, cancer cells have more membranes and individual cells are more closely packed than surrounding normal prostatic tissue. This results in restricted diffusion of water molecules and higher signal intensity of cancer cells relative to a normal gland. Both these MRI techniques may help improve the currently modest staging accuracy of MRI. There is also recent interest in the use of pre-biopsy MRI of the prostate for risk stratification prior to biopsy and identification of the index focus of prostate cancer for targeted focal therapy.

Reference

Abuzallouf S, Dayes I, Lukka H. Baseline staging of newly diagnosed prostate cancer: a summary of the literature. *J Urol* 2004;**171**:2122–7.

Further reading

Hricak H, Choyke P, Eberhardt S et al. Imaging prostate cancer: a multidisciplinary perspective. *Radiology* 2007;**243**:28–53.

Husband J, Sohaib A. Prostate cancer. In Hushand J, Resnek R (eds) *Imaging in oncology*. London: Informa Healthcare, 2004.

NICE Clinical Guideline 58, *Prostate Cancer, Diagnosis and Treatment*. February 2008. (http://guidance.nice.org.uk/CG58).

Prostate Cancer Risk Management Programme. Undertaking a transrectal ultrasound guided biopsy of the prostate. 2006. (www.cancerscreening.nhs.uk/prostate/pcrmp01.pdf).

CHAPTER 6

Screening for Prostate Cancer

Richard J. Bryant and Freddie C. Hamdy

Nuffield Department of Surgical Sciences, University of Oxford, Oxford, UK

OVERVIEW

- Screening describes the diagnosis of pre-clinical cases of a significant condition at an early stage in order to reduce harm from the disease
- Several requirements are essential to justify a prostate cancer mass screening programme
- PSA-based prostate cancer screening has substantial limitations
- PSA-testing causes over-diagnosis and over-treatment of clinically insignificant prostate cancer
- There is currently insufficient evidence of benefit from PSA-based prostate cancer screening to justify its introduction as a public health policy

---

Table 6.1 Requirements of a screening programme.

- The disease is an important health problem
- The natural history of the disease is well understood
- The disease is recognizable at an early stage
- Treatment at an early stage is better
- A suitable diagnostic test exists
- An acceptable test exists
- Adequate facilities exist to deal with abnormalities detected
- Screening is done at repeated intervals when the onset is insidious
- The chance of harm from screening is less than the chance of benefit
- The cost of screening is balanced against the benefits.

Introduction

Prostate cancer screening is a continuing controversial issue. Until recently most reviews of the available scientific evidence concluded that routine population screening could not be recommended because of the lack of evidence that this would improve either survival or the quality of men's lives. However, recent data from the European Randomized study of Screening for Prostate Cancer (ERSPC) provide for the first time evidence that screening using PSA testing can reduce mortality from the disease by approximately 20% in populations of men at risk between the ages of 55 and 69 years, and a more recent subgroup analysis suggests a higher rate of mortality reduction. However, many concerns surround these new data. In the United Kingdom, the current approach is to provide men with sufficient information regarding PSA testing to enable them to make an informed decision about undergoing this test rather than to introduce mass screening for prostate cancer.

Principles of screening

Screening is the diagnosis of a disease during its asymptomatic stage within a population at risk using a suitable test. The aim of screening is to reduce the mortality of a disease by diagnosing it at an earlier stage when radical treatment has a greater chance of cure than awaiting a later clinical diagnosis. Prostate cancer can be diagnosed at a pre-clinical stage through PSA testing and prostate biopsy. Localised prostate cancer can be treated and cured by surgery or different forms of radiotherapy. For a disease to be suitable for screening, a number of criteria need to be considered (Table 6.1).

The disease should be an important health problem

Prostate cancer is the commonest male malignancy in the Western world and the second leading cause of male cancer-related death. In the United Kingdom, in 2006, 35,515 men were diagnosed with prostate cancer and 10,168 men died from the disease. Prostate cancer incidence rose during the 1990s due to PSA testing. In some countries, mortality rates from prostate cancer has decreased, but while some of these reductions may be attributable to PSA testing, the decline in mortality occurred too soon after PSA testing was introduced for this effect to be completely attributable to screening (Figure 6.1). There is little doubt that prostate cancer represents a significant public health burden in Western countries.

The natural history of the disease should be well understood

Clinically detected prostate cancer may progress very slowly, but the natural history of screen-detected prostate cancer is less well understood. 'Clinically significant' prostate cancers are by definition

ABC of Prostate Cancer, First Edition.
Edited by Prokar Dasgupta and Roger S. Kirby.
© 2012 Blackwell Publishing Ltd. Published 2012 by Blackwell Publishing Ltd.

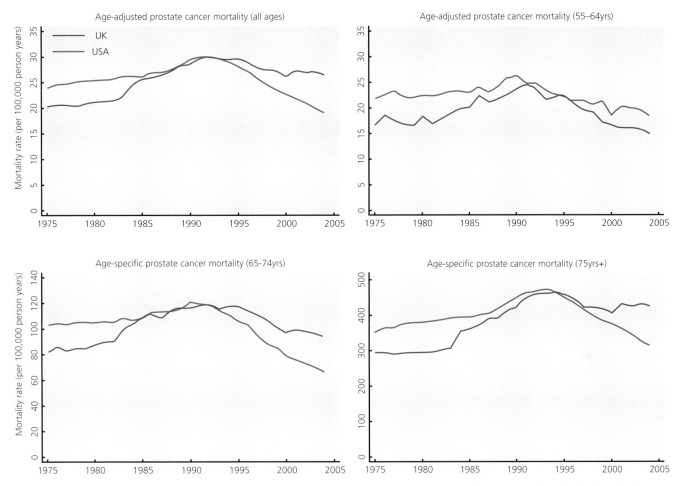

Figure 6.1 US and UK prostate cancer mortality rates 1975–2004. Reproduced from Lancet Oncology 2008;**9**(5):445–452 with permission from Elsevie.

at risk of progression and may, if not detected through screening or case-finding, become lethal. The majority of screen-detected prostate cancer may never become clinically significant, and many men will therefore die of other competing causes. The 'lead time' is the time by which the date of diagnosis is advanced through screening rather than clinical detection and is around 5–10 years for prostate cancer. As screening would predominantly detect low-risk localised prostate cancer, it is important to distinguish 'clinically significant' cases, which require treatment, from 'indolent' cases, which may be managed conservatively. Many PSA-detected prostate cancers may therefore be 'over-treated' with adverse effects on quality of life and no evidence of improvement in survival.

There should be effective treatments for the disease

Men with localised prostate cancer have numerous curative treatment options, or may undergo active surveillance for 'low-risk' disease. There is, however, little robust randomised trial data comparing the efficacy of treatment options for screen-detected localised prostate cancer. A Scandinavian randomised study showed that in clinically detected prostate cancer, radical prostatectomy reduced disease-specific mortality by 50% and progression by 40% compared with 'watchful waiting', but this may not be applicable to

screen-detected disease. In the UK, ProtecT (Prostate Testing for Cancer and Treatment) is a randomised controlled trial of treatment effectiveness in men with clinically localised prostate comparing active monitoring, surgery and radiotherapy in PSA-detected prostate cancer. The study is supported by HTA NIHR and results are awaited. Despite the current use of serum PSA and Gleason grading, it can be difficult to accurately risk stratify localised prostate cancer as 'indolent' or potentially aggressive. Novel molecular biology techniques may accurately differentiate these cases and improve the accuracy with which men are directed towards treatment.

Screening tests should be acceptable

Ideal screening tests are safe and acceptable and have a high sensitivity, specificity, positive predicative value and negative predictive value. PSA testing compromises between sensitivity and specificity as demonstrated by the observation that if the PSA threshold for a biopsy is reduced from 4 ng/ml to 2 ng/ml, more prostate cancers are detected but more negative biopsies are performed. A 'positive' PSA result does not always signify the presence of a prostate cancer while there is no true low limit of PSA that excludes prostate cancer. The ERSPC trial biopsied those men with a PSA above 3 ng/ml, but the ideal PSA-threshold for screening is not defined. The screening interval (between 1–4 years) and ages at which screening should occur also need clarification. Elderly men with a short life expectancy, or younger men with significant co-morbidity, should not undergo screening as they are unlikely to experience any benefit and could be harmed. It is also important to realise that prostate cancer screening involves a PSA test followed by a prostate biopsy if the PSA is raised, therefore a consideration of the acceptability of screening must also take into account the biopsy procedure itself, which is not without morbidity and side-effects.

Adequate facilities should be available to manage abnormalities detected

Men with an elevated PSA are usually invited to undergo a prostate biopsy, and if this detects prostate cancer, staging and grading of the disease are used to guide treatment options. Although around 20–25% of men with an elevated PSA are found to have prostate cancer on the first biopsy, there is a significant false negative rate. The biopsy may reveal abnormal pathology such as high-grade prostatic intraepithelial neoplasia (PIN) or atypical small acinar proliferation (ASAP). A screening programme would need to provide adequate guidance regarding the necessity of repeat biopsies in these scenarios, and new molecular diagnostic tests such as urinary PCA3 levels may be used to reduce unnecessary repeat testing.

The chance of benefit should exceed the risk of harm

Screening aims to reduce disease-specific morbidity and mortality and increase quality of life but there is the possibility that numerous adverse effects may occur (Table 6.2). Screening may detect 'indolent' prostate cancer posing little or no threat but the patient may be 'over-treated' resulting in impotence or urinary incontinence. It is imperative that any evaluation of prostate cancer screening assesses quality-of-life issues.

Two large trials of prostate cancer screening have recently reported their results (Table 6.3). The ERSPC trial demonstrates that screening reduces mortality by 27% at a median follow-up of 9 years but a 'number needed to treat' analysis reveals that 1410 men need to undergo PSA-testing and 48 men need treatment in order to save one life. More recently, a subgroup analysis of the Swedish cohort with longer follow-up suggested that the reduction in mortality was 44%, with number needed to screen and treat

Table 6.2 Effects of prostate cancer screening.

Favourable	Unfavourable
Life-years gained	Attendance for screening
Prostate cancer-related deaths prevented	Screen-detected false positive PSA results and unnecessary biopsies
Reduced number of prostate biopsies with a negative result outside of the screening programme	Increase in life-years after diagnosis without improved survival (lead-time bias)
Prevention of advanced prostate cancer	Additional radical treatments and 'over-treatment'
	False reassurance of a negative result

Table 6.3 Summary of evidence from the two largest trials of screening.

	ERSPC	PCLO
Setting	7 European centres	United States of America
Age	55–69 years	55–74 years
Number of men	162,243	76,693
PSA threshold for biopsy	3 ng/ml	4 ng/ml
Follow-up	9 years	7 years
Outcome	20% improvement in survival of screened versus non-screened individuals	No difference in survival of screened versus non-screened individuals

reduced to 293 and 12 respectively. Confirmation of these findings is awaited from the larger ERSPC cohort. The Prostate, Lung, Colorectal and Ovary cancer screening trial in the USA reported no significant improvement in survival but this negative result may partly be explained by the fact that over half of the participants in the control group were contaminated by PSA testing. At present, the adoption of population screening for prostate cancer as a public health policy is unjustified due to the large over-treatment effect demonstrated. Before the introduction of screening is considered by healthcare providers as a public health policy, the level of current opportunistic screening, over-diagnosis, over-treatment, quality of life issues, costs, and cost-effectiveness of existing treatments should be taken into account.

Future developments

'Targeted screening' may accurately detect 'clinically significant' prostate cancer, resulting in a more effective screening programme for this disease. The use of single nucleotide polymorphism (SNP) analysis, for example, may enable improved targeting of men potentially harbouring 'clinically significant' disease. The ERSPC has demonstrated that screening reduces the detection of locally advanced and metastatic prostate cancer. This in itself could be used as a powerful argument for the introduction of screening, but not before we improve methods of discriminating men who are at risk of having significant prostate cancer *before* the diagnosis, and those *with* the diagnosis of early disease who can be kept safely within a window of curability through refined active monitoring protocols, novel panels of biomarkers and reliable risk calculators.

Conclusion

Prostate cancer screening remains controversial. Current published data do not justify implementing prostate cancer screening based on PSA testing, as stated recently by the NHS Prostate Cancer Risk Management Programme. Future efforts should be directed at targeting screening towards men at high risk of 'clinically significant' disease who will benefit from treatment, possibly using genetic markers. This warrants urgent translational research for the development of novel prognostic biomarkers and reliable risk calculators.

Further reading

Andriole GL et al. Mortality results from a randomized prostate-cancer screening trial. *N Engl J Med* 2009;**360**(13):1310–19.

Collin SM et al. Prostate-cancer mortality in the USA and UK in 1975–2004: An ecological study. *Lancet Oncology* 2008;**9**(5):445–52.

Hugosson J, Carlsson S, Aus G et al. Mortality results from the Göteborg randomised population-based prostate-cancer screening trial. *Lancet Oncology* 2010;**11**(8):725–32.

Lane JA, Hamdy FC, Martin RM, Turner EL, Neal DE, Donovan JL. Latest results from the UK trials evaluating prostate cancer screening and treatment: The CAP and ProtecT studies. *Eur J Cancer* 2010;**46**(17): 3095–101.

Schröder FH et al. Screening and prostate-cancer mortality in a randomized European study. *N Engl J Med* 2009;**360**(13):1320–8.

CHAPTER 7

Active Surveillance

Judith Dockray[1], Pardeep Kumar[2], Lars Holmberg[1] and Gordon Muir[1]

[1]King's College London, UK
[2]Guy's and St Thomas' Hospital NHS Foundation Trust, London, UK

OVERVIEW

- Active surveillance (AS) is a management option in prostate cancer, the primary aim of which is to avoid unnecessary treatment in men with indolent cancers

- AS is an intervention undergoing evaluation and awaiting level one evidence from randomised control trials (RCTs) for safety and quality of care to support its use

- AS is an option for carefully selected low risk patients who are candidates for curative intervention should clinical parameters indicate that the disease is no longer indolent

- In general, AS protocols require regular clinical examination, PSA testing and repeat prostate biopsy

- Limited published follow-up is available for patients on AS protocols, the results of several RCTS are awaited

Introduction

According to Cancer Research UK (2010), prostate cancer (CaP) is the most common cancer in men in the UK. However, it is clear that a significant proportion of patients diagnosed with CaP will never develop symptoms nor see a reduction in their life expectancy due to the disease. In addition, we know that treatments for CaP may actually cause significant morbidity, including urinary incontinence, erectile dysfunction and an increase in cardiovascular morbidity. It is therefore vital that intervention for CaP is offered in a timely fashion to those who will benefit while treatment is deferred in those who will not. Some statistics on prostate cancer risks are:

- The lifetime risk of dying from CaP is 1 in 33.
- The risk of a man over 50 years of age being diagnosed with CaP is 1 in 6.
- The risk of a man over 50 years of age having histological evidence of CaP is 1 in 3 (on autopsy).

It can be inferred from these figures that the incidence to mortality ratio is almost 8:1. It could be argued that this corresponds to a degree of over-diagnosis, i.e. patients being diagnosed with CaP when the disease will not affect them clinically nor shorten their life span.

What is active surveillance?

Active surveillance (AS) is a methodology of patient monitoring with the primary aim of avoiding unnecessary treatment in men with indolent cancers. Follow-up ideally identifies those patients who have progressive cancers at a stage where intervention will still be curative. It is therefore indicated in those who have potentially curable disease but do not require this at the time of diagnosis or in those who wish to defer intervention for as long as is safe, with the aim of avoiding the complications of intervention. It may also be used as part of a treatment strategy in those who intend to undergo curative treatment but wish to defer this for a period of time until circumstances allow.

Why is active surveillance an option in prostate cancer?

From 1990–2002, the annual age-adjusted incidence of prostate cancer increased twofold. This increase was largely due to PSA testing enabling the detection of low-grade, low-volume ($<0.5\,\text{cm}^3$) and impalpable disease in asymptomatic men. This corresponds to considerable lead-time bias, reported as between 9.9–13.3 years, as tumours are diagnosed well before they may become clinically relevant. Although the natural history of prostate cancer is heterogeneous, and not fully understood, it has been argued that around 60% of these men would not experience clinically significant progression during their lifespan due to age at diagnosis, competing co-morbidities or low-grade tumour status. Active surveillance aims to identify this group who will not develop clinically significant disease, sparing them the morbidity of over-treatment, while identifying those in whom disease progression is likely.

What is the difference between active surveillance and watchful waiting?

Watchful waiting is an approach usually employed in elderly men with significant co-morbidity who are asymptomatic. It is the

ABC of Prostate Cancer, First Edition.
Edited by Prokar Dasgupta and Roger S. Kirby.
© 2012 Blackwell Publishing Ltd. Published 2012 by Blackwell Publishing Ltd.

postponement of therapy (usually hormone manipulation) until symptoms occur with the intention to palliate CaP rather than attempt to cure it, as with active surveillance.

How is active surveillance undertaken?

The inclusion of AS in the National Institute for Clinical Excellence (NICE) guidelines (2008) infers that there is consensus on the method of AS when, in actual fact, none exists. AS is an intervention undergoing evaluation and awaiting level one evidence from randomised control trials for safety and quality of care to support its use.

The common features of the differing protocols include:

- regular physical examination (including digital rectal examination, DRE);
- regular serum PSA;
- repeat prostate biopsies.

The ideal interval between investigations is unknown and is the subject of current study. A typical regime would involve three-monthly PSA estimations, six-monthly DREs and repeat prostate biopsy at between one and two years after initial diagnosis. This regime would continue in those who remain stable with no evidence of clinical, biochemical or histological progression. Around 10% of patients opt out of active surveillance programmes out of choice, unwilling to live with the perceived degree of uncertainty this type of monitoring incurs.

What is the evidence for active surveillance?

If we extrapolate data from patient groups from the pre-PSA era, a significant proportion with low-grade, low-volume disease who are initially identified by PSA screening alone will have a longer than 20-year disease-specific survival with no treatment. Current data support this hypothesis but, however, are derived from non-mature randomised controlled trials with follow-up of less than 10 years. These AS studies in patients with CaP (predominantly identified by PSA screening rather than those presenting with symptoms or abnormal clinical examination) consistently show low rates of tumour progression and high rates of disease-specific survival (10-year CaP specific survival rates of 99–100%). In the same studies, the proportion of patients opting out of AS protocols to undergo intervention ranges from 14–31%. However, the median range of follow-up in these patients is 24–64 months and longer-term data are awaited. Several international studies are under way, including Standard Treatment against Restricted Treatment (START), Prostate Testing for Cancer and Treatment (ProTeCT), Prostate Cancer Intervention Versus Observation Trial (PIVOT) and Prostate cancer Research International: Active Surveillance (PRIAS).

For which patients is active surveillance an option?

Serum PSA, tumour grade and tumour volume may be used to predict risk of progression of CaP. Current nomograms (of which

Table 7.1 Risk categories for CaP-specific progression at 10 years.

Risk	Clinical stage	PSA	Gleason score
Low risk	T1a-T2a	<10 ng/ml	2–6
Intermediate risk	T2b-T2c	10–20 ng/ml	7
High risk	T3a	>20	8–10

there are at least 40 published variants) tend to be based upon follow-up of patients who have undergone radical intervention for CaP, usually radical prostatectomy, as tumour grade and volume can be reliably measured in this group. However, the tools presently available provide a guide only and must be tailored to the individual.

The majority of guidelines on active surveillance use the risk stratification parameters described by D'Amico and colleagues which have been validated in patients undergoing both radical prostatectomy and radical radiotherapy. Each risk category describes the risk of CaP-specific progression at 10 years (Table 7.1).

Both the American and European Urology Associations recommend that active surveillance is discussed with low and intermediate risk prostate cancer patients. In 2008, NICE produced guidelines on the diagnosis and treatment of CaP. Active surveillance was recommended as first-line treatment for men with low-risk CaP. In response to concerns raised by UK urologists and oncologists due to the lack of long-term data on this treatment option, a joint NICE and British Association of Urological Surgeons (BAUS) statement was subsequently issued, confirming that all management options should be discussed with low risk patients.

Several other variables are considered in addition to the clinical stage, PSA and tumour grade. These depend upon the AS protocol employed and include:

- the percentage of positive cores taken at trans-rectal guided prostate biopsy and percentage of maximal core involved with prostate cancer;
- PSA kinetics – including the estimated time for the PSA to double (doubling time) vs. PSA velocity and percentage of maximal core involvement (<50%);
- PSA density (the PSA normalised for prostate volume estimated with trans-rectal ultrasound);
- patients must be fully motivated to participate and understand that follow-up visits are mandatory in order not to miss possible tumour progression.

Benefits of active surveillance

AS is attractive to patients due to the lack of side-effects associated with curative treatment options. Many men with low-volume, low-grade disease will never need treatment, and elderly men will often die of another medical condition before their prostate cancer manifests clinically.

Potential risks of active surveillance

Determining which men are at greatest risk of disease progression is challenging. Most centres operate on a combination of Gleason grade, PSA and clinical stage. There are currently studies comparing the velocity of PSA rise with PSA doubling time and considerable debate still arises as to which is the most accurate predictor of progression.

As the prostate cancer is not actually being treated, there is always the possibility of disease progression that could ultimately lead to death. A more advanced stage of disease at a later date may have limited treatment options open to the patient with more unpalatable side-effects. Careful selection of patients onto an active surveillance programme is vital. Patients must be highly motivated and prepared for the degree of commitment that entering into an active surveillance programme entails.

There is also the degree of psychological stresses that occurs due to the knowledge of being diagnosed with cancer without actually being treated for it. A proportion of patients find this unacceptable and decline AS for this reason. Studies have shown that having dedicated nurses for this patient group significantly decreases this anxiety by providing the reassurance of having easy access back into medical care.

When to identify that the disease has progressed?

Identifying significant disease progression is the key to successful AS and the ability to offer radical treatment while the condition is still curable. Many different regimes have been published and there continues to be a lack of cohesion in deciding an appropriate regime. Most agree that the following are important:

- change in DRE;
- rising PSA – either PSA velocity or doubling time. CaPSURE demonstrated this was the greatest trigger for active treatment. However, the randomised control trial from the Scandinavian Prostate Cancer Study Group showed that it was unsafe to use PSA kinetics in isolation as a marker to exclude disease progression.
- increased Gleason grade;
- increased tumour volume on biopsy, though the debate as to which is most reliable of standard trans-rectal biopsy versus trans-perineal template and saturation biopsies remains.

The role of serial imaging is under investigation.

The decision to progress from AS to radical treatment should be made with the patient and based on co-morbidities, life expectancy and personal preference.

Future directions

There has been considerable interest in the use of novel biomarkers for predicting the behaviour of individual tumours, e.g. TMPRSS2:ERG gene fusion, which may predict a more aggressive disease phenotype. Gene signatures including gains 11q13.1 and deletions 8p23.2 have been shown to predict PSA recurrences post prostatectomy, irrespective of grade and stage of primary tumour.

Conclusion

Active surveillance is an alternative to immediate treatment of localised prostate cancer in men with presumed low-risk disease. Cancer registry data suggest that active surveillance is a currently under-utilised treatment option. This is in part due to concerns of missing clinically significant disease progression. Medium-term studies seem to confirm that in carefully selected men, delayed treatment does not appear to compromise outcomes for these patients, however, prospective studies of AS entry criteria are required in order to standardise the definition of 'low-risk'. Long-term data from studies such as ProTeCT, START, PIVOT and PRIAS are awaited.

Further reading

AUA Guidelines for the Management of Clinically Localised Prostate Cancer, 2007. (www.auanet.org).

Bastian, PJ et al. Insignificant prostate cancer and active surveillance: From definition to clinical implications. *European Urology* 2009;**55**:1321–32.

Dall'Era MA et al. Active surveillance for early-stage prostate cancer. *Cancer* 2008;**112**(8):1650–9.

EAU Guidelines on Prostate Cancer, 2010. (www.uroweb.org).

NICE Clinical Guideline 58, *Prostate Cancer, Diagnosis and Treatment*. February 2008. (http://guidance.nice.org.uk/CG58).

Weissbach L, Altwein J. Active surveillance or active treatment in localised prostate cancer? *J. Deutsches Artzeblatt International* 2009;**106**(22):371–6.

Wilt, TJ, Thompson, IM. Clinically localised prostate cancer. *BMJ* 2006;**333**: 1102–6.

CHAPTER 8

Open Radical Prostatectomy

Wim van Haute[1] and Hein van Poppel[2]

[1]Department of Urology, St Rembert Hospital, Torhout; St Jan Hospital, Bruges, Belgium
[2]Department of Urology, Katholieke Universiteit, University Hospital Gasthuisberg, Leuven, Belgium

---

OVERVIEW

- Indications for radical prostatectomy
- Decision-making using determining factors
- Pre- and post-operative care
- Description of the surgical technique
- The most frequent and important complications

Introduction

Radical surgical removal of the prostate has become the gold standard in the treatment of localised prostate cancer. Although radical prostatectomy (RP) only became widely adopted in the mid-1980s, the first radical perineal prostatectomy was performed over a century ago by the French surgeon Proust in 1901. However, most historical reviews will mention H. Young as the first to describe this procedure at the Johns Hopkins University. Millin was the first to describe a retropubic approach to the prostate, and the retrograde radical prostatectomy was first described by Chute, and a few years later by Campbell.

The procedure remained very unpopular because of the high morbidity and blood loss, while it was often treating a cancer that was not life-threatening. Only later, with the study of the anatomy of the dorsal vein complex (DVC) and the neurovascular bundles (NVB) by Dr P. Walsh, together with the widespread application of PSA testing, has radical prostatectomy become more popular.

Indications

Radical prostatectomy has been shown to give the best long-term chance of cure from localised early prostate cancer. It is now considered the best way to eradicate organ-confined disease and selected cases of locally advanced disease. Disease-related factors, but also patient-related factors are important.

ABC of Prostate Cancer, First Edition.
Edited by Prokar Dasgupta and Roger S. Kirby.
© 2012 Blackwell Publishing Ltd. Published 2012 by Blackwell Publishing Ltd.

Disease-related factors

In the treatment choice, PSA value, TNM stage, Gleason score and estimated tumour volume have to be considered. In the AUA and EAU guidelines, RP is recommended for T1 and T2 tumours, when life expectancy is good. EAU guidelines do recommend watchful waiting for T1a tumours in older men. The British Association of Urologists (BAUS) has issued wider indications for watchful waiting. Until recently, T3 disease was considered advanced, and urologists were reluctant to perform surgery. Now most guidelines agree on cT3 as a surgical disease in well-selected patients, and in multimodal treatment.

Patient-related factors

Age

Age at diagnosis is considered a strong predictive factor of cure of disease. Studies show a better long-term cancer control after radical prostatectomy in patients aged under 50.

In many centres, radical prostatectomy is advised up to 75 years of age, and for men with a life expectancy of at least ten years. Life expectancy, however, has to be regarded as a more important factor than age.

Surgical risk

It is important to do a thorough check-up on the general health status and co-morbidities in every patient to assess the surgical risk, and the risk–benefit ratio. It has to be mentioned that obesity is an important factor, not only for the direct surgical risk due to a more difficult procedure, but a higher BMI is related to higher grade disease, more extraprostatic extension, and more positive surgical margins. Obesity can be a reason for preferring open radical prostatectomy over laparoscopic or robotic procedures, because of the higher anaesthetic risks of the necessary Trendelenburg position in the latter approaches.

Surgical technique

Pre-operative preparation

After having diagnosed prostate cancer on a trans-rectal ultrasound (TRUS) guided biopsy, it is best to wait a couple of weeks before proceeding to radical prostatectomy. In the case of transurethral resection of the prostate (TURP), one should wait 12 weeks at least. Both procedures cause an inflammatory effect, and possible haematoma, which could make it more difficult to find the correct anatomical planes during the radical prostatectomy and so raise the chance of surgical complications, such as rectal injury. They also render more difficult the evaluation of possible extraprostatic extension, or the preservation of the neurovascular bundle. Pre-operatively, the decision has to be made whether a nerve-sparing procedure will be attempted, taking localisation, grade, extent, and the finding of digital rectal examination, TRUS and/or MRI into consideration.

An important factor in the preparation for surgery is the colon preparation although some experts no longer advocate this. A clean and empty colon is important both for surgical access, and in case of a rectal injury, to avoid massive contamination of the surgical field.

Anaesthesia

Nowadays most centres prefer a combined spinal-epidural anaesthetic instead of a general anaesthetic. Studies show that this approach gives less peroperative blood loss, quicker recovery, and less post-operative pain. Reports suggest that there is less chance of deep venous thrombosis and pulmonary embolism.

Procedure

The patient is placed in a supine position, with slight flex on the table, and some Trendelenburg to give better access to the pelvis. At the beginning of the procedure, a catheter of ≥20 French is inserted.

Depending on the centre, incision can be midline sub-umbilical, which is most common. A Pfannenstiel incision can be helpful if a hernia has to be repaired, but tends to be less satisfactory to reach the deep pelvis. Radical prostatectomy is performed extra-peritoneally so the pre-peritoneal space of Retzius is opened. By gentle cephalad retraction of the bladder and sweeping off fatty tissue, the anterior aspect of the prostate end the endopelvic fascia are exposed. If necessary, a limited or extended lymph node dissection is carried out at this stage of the procedure.

Incision of the endopelvic fascia is done on both sides; this has to be done on the levator ani muscle laterally, in order not to damage the dorsal vein complex (DVC) (or Santorini's plexus). Next, the puboprostatic ligaments are divided to get access to the apex of the prostate and the overlying venous complex of Santorini (Figure 8.1).

By palpation, the plane between Santorini's and the urethra is identified, and a large distal ligation stitch of the DVC is placed. A second suture is placed at the base of the prostate to prevent back bleeding. Now the DVC can be divided by electrocautery or sharp dissection. Any bleeding from the DVC is over-sewn at this stage.

Next, by gentle blunt dissection, very close to the urethra, the NVB are separated from the prostatic apex. A right-angled clamp is passed under the urethra, to avoid rectal injury, and the urethra is divided by sharp dissection. At this stage, some urologists insert some urethral stitches for the later anastomosis.

The apical dissection is a critical manoeuvre in the procedure, first of all because of the close relation to the NVB, but also because it has to be resected completely to avoid apical positive margins.

Next, the posterior aspect of the prostate is bluntly dissected with the index finger. At this stage, depending on the indication

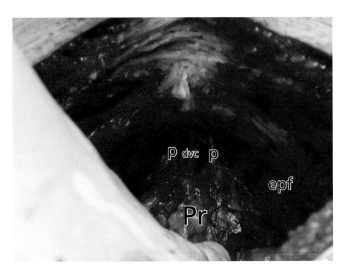

Figure 8.1 View on anterior side of Prostate (Pr). P, puboprostatic ligament; dvc, superficial dorsal vein complex; EPF, opened endopelvic fascia.

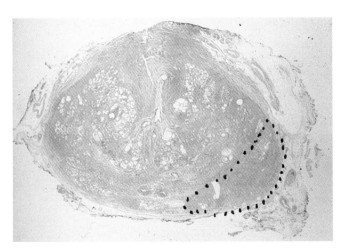

Figure 8.2 Transsectional view of prostate specimen. Dotted zone is the tumor, covered by the resected NVB, the other side is nerve sparing.

of a nerve-sparing or non-nerve-sparing procedure, the NVB is either taken along with the prostate, or the lateral dissection is done closely to the prostate, without touching the NVB (Figure 8.2).

Now the dorsal dissection is extended cranially towards the seminal vesicles (SV), with excision of Denonvillier's fascia along with the prostate. The SV are then dissected, the artery at the tip of the vesicle is clipped and the vas deferens is transsected.

The bladder neck can either be spared or resected (Figure 8.3). In the latter case, a racket reconstruction is performed with careful avoidance of the ureteral orifices.

Now the prostate is fully resected, and the specimen is checked for capsular incision. If an incision is found, an extra resection can be done at the corresponding location.

Meticulous hemostasis is done, avoiding the use of electrocautery in the case of a nerve-sparing procedure (Figure 8.4). Anastomosis between the bladder neck and the urethral stump is performed with 4 or 6 seperate stitches. A 3-0 monofilament resorbable thread is used.

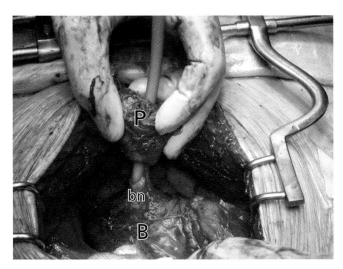

Figure 8.3 Bladder neck sparing prostatectomy: B, bladder, P, prostate; bn, bladder neck.

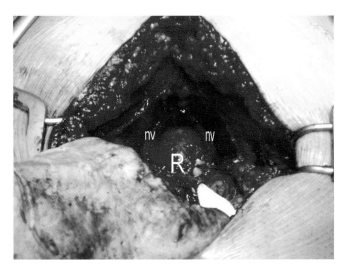

Figure 8.4 View of pelvis post resection and hemostasis. Nv, neurovascular bundle; R, rectum.

The last step of the procedure is the vesico-urethral anastomosis. After placing a 16F Foley catheter, four sutures are placed at 2, 5 7 and 10 o'clock. The bladder comes down and the sutures are tied while traction is applied on the inflated balloon catheter.

The anastomosis is checked for leakage, and two suction drains are placed in the pelvis. The abdomen is closed in layers, with staples on the skin.

Post-operative care

After radical prostatectomy, there is no need for intensive care hospitalisation. Pain control is perfect with a patient controlled analgesia (PCA) pump, which is left in situ for two days.

The main points of interest post-operatively are general status, wound control, drain volume and bowel movements. As soon as peristalsis is restored, feeding starts gradually, mostly on the second post-operative day. Drains are removed when daily production is less than 10 ml.

To prevent thrombo-embolism, low molecular weight heparin is started according to patient weight and risk factors and is best continued for 35 days.

Median hospital stay after open radical prostatectomy is 4–6 days. The urethral catheter stays in situ for about 10 days, after which it can be removed. A cystogram is only done before removal if any post-operative problem has occurred that might cause leakage. Immediately after removal of the catheter, pelvic floor exercises are started, to improve continence.

Complications

Early complications

There are conventional perioperative or early post-operative complications such as wound infection, post-operative ileus, DVT and pulmonary embolism. More specifically, after radical prostatectomy, post-operative bleeding is not a rare event. It is mostly caused by bleeding of the DVC, but also in nerve-sparing procedures, there is a higher blood loss. This will only rarely exceed 1000 ml.

Rectal injury is also a possibility during this procedure, but a temporary protective colostomy is only very rarely indicated. When, however, a urethrorectal fistula occurs, an immediate colostomy is mandatory. Previous TURP or rectal surgery gives a higher chance of rectal injury.

Dehiscence of the anastomosis almost only occurs after unfortunate accidental withdrawal of an inflated balloon catheter. Conservative management with a prolonged, correctly placed indwelling catheter is mandatory.

Late complications

The specific long-term complications of radical prostatectomy are incontinence, erectile dysfunction and urethral stricture.

Incontinence

For most patients, this is the most disabling complication. The incidence varies from 3–30%, according to the literature. In experienced hands it is less than 10%. More than 90% of patients regain continence in the first year, and 95% of patients are satisfied with the degree of incontinence. Pelvic floor exercises, eventually started before surgery, are helpful.

Erectile dysfunction

The degree of erectile dysfunction depends mainly on the quality of the nerve-sparing procedure. Even if NVB is spared, elongation (neurotmesis) of the nerve occurs and re-enervation will take about 8–9 months. Depending on age, the recovery is about 60–75% for patients under 60, dropping to 45–50% for patients over 65.

Starting PDE-5 inhibitors early could improve the recovery of the erectile function. Some experts will advocate an early start of self-injection therapy.

Anastomotic stricture

In 0.5–9% of cases, anastomotic stricture occurs. The incidence is higher if previous TURP has been performed, or if the bladder neck is resected. Initial treatment with urethral dilatation can be quite successful but sometimes repeated endoscopic procedures, compromising urinary continence, can be necessary.

Further reading

Heidenreich A, Aus G, Bolla M, et al. EAU guidelines on prostate cancer. *Actas Urol Esp* 2009;**33**(2):113–26.

Hsu CY, Joniau S, Van Poppel H. *Radical prostatectomy for locally advanced prostate cancer: Technical aspects of radical prostatectomy*. EAU update series 3 2005:90–7.

Van Poppel H, Hsu CY, Joniau S. Indications for radical prostatectomy. In: *Radical Prostatectomy: from open to robotic*. Eds.: Roger Kirby, Francesco Montorsi, Joseph A. Smith, Paolo Gontero, 2007:23–27.

CHAPTER 9

Laparoscopic Radical Prostatectomy

Pardeep Kumar and Declan Cahill

Guy's and St Thomas' Hospital NHS Foundation Trust, London, UK

OVERVIEW

- Radical prostatectomy is the gold standard treatment for organ-confined prostate cancer
- Surgery can be achieved safely and with excellent outcomes using laparoscopic techniques
- Patients must understand the risks of post-operative incontinence and erectile dysfunction. These can be minimised by pre-operative counselling, operative technique and post-operative rehabilitation therapy
- Laparoscopic radical prostatectomy should be performed in high volume centres where training and mentorship can ensure high quality outcomes while optimising learning curves.
- Continuous audit enables early identification of problems and facilitates improved outcomes. Run charts detailing consecutive patients are useful

---

Introduction

The key outcome measures for radical prostatectomy are oncological control of CaP with preservation of sexual function and urinary continence. The aim is to achieve these measures safely with as little suffering and discomfort for the patient as possible within the financial constraints of the providing healthcare system.

Advantages of laparoscopy

The magnification used in laparoscopy offers high definition exposure of the pelvic organs without the trauma of access of open surgery. In addition, it allows precise identification of fascial planes and structures such as the neurovascular bundles which lie alongside the prostate, vital in preserving sexual function and continence. An accurate vesico-urethral anastamosis is facilitated by laparoscopy. The pneumoperitoneum provides the space and the positive pressure to limit low pressure blood loss. Tactile feedback is maintained in laparoscopy and is yet to be reproduced using the robotic platform.

History of laparoscopic radical prostatectomy

Laparoscopic radical prostatectomy (LRP) was first described by Schuessler et al. in 1997. LRP has been performed in and exported by the Institut Mutualiste Montsouris, Paris, since January 1998 under the stewardship of Professor Guy Vallancien. This technique was initially disseminated throughout Europe where the benefits of laparoscopy have been embraced for many years. LRP has been refined with improved imaging and surgical equipment and a constant drive to improve outcomes from surgeon to surgeon, institution to institution and from technique to technique. It is from the seed of laparoscopic radical prostatectomy and the challenges it posed to open surgery, along with opportunity it gave to robotic surgery that so much of the improvement in outcome of radical prostatectomy has come.

Patient selection

Patients are selected for surgery on the basis of several factors. These can broadly be divided into disease-specific and patient-specific factors.

Disease-specific factors

Is the CaP organ confined? This decision is based on the following items:

- pre-treatment PSA
- digital rectal examination
- grade and volume of disease on prostate biopsy
- staging examinations (MRI and bone scan where appropriate).

Patient-specific factors

Is the patient fit for surgery and will he benefit from an attempt at curing CaP which, in some cases, may only become clinically apparent 10 years after diagnosis? The decision is based on the following factors:

- age
- fitness and performance status
- co-morbidities

ABC of Prostate Cancer, First Edition.
Edited by Prokar Dasgupta and Roger S. Kirby.
© 2012 Blackwell Publishing Ltd. Published 2012 by Blackwell Publishing Ltd.

- previous pelvic surgery or radiotherapy
- willingness to accept surgical intervention and usual postoperative course as well as possible complications.

The above factors are taken into account with every patient. To optimise outcomes, CaP treatment must be tailored to the individual. For some men, surgery is unacceptable. For others, having complete removal of a cancerous organ is the only option. Specific anaesthetic contra-indications for laparoscopic surgery are high intra-cranial pressure and severe cardio-pulmonary disease.

Surgical challenges include obese patients, big prostates, a small bony pelvis, middle lobes, the need for nerve-sparing or wide local excision (highest risk of rectal injury), previous TURP and previous abdominal surgery including extraperitoneal hernia mesh placement.

Operative details

Position

The patient is placed supine with the legs abducted to allow for access to the rectum and closer placement of the monitor. The patient is draped and pressure points are protected. Transperitoneal surgery requires an exaggerated Trendelenberg (head down) position whereas in extraperitoneal surgery the patient may be almost supine.

Port placement

Port placement varies from surgeon to surgeon and is dependent upon the patient's anatomy, namely the distance between umbilicus and symphisis pubis and width of the true pelvis. Five ports are usually used. A 10 mm umbilical camera port, three 5 mm ports and a 10 mm port. Two surgical ports in each of the left and right iliac fossa with the 10 mm port placed according to preference for the needle driver and 10 mm instrument access (Figure 9.1).

The surgeon stands to the left of the patient, the assistant on the right, both facing the feet of the patient. Ideally, a robotic system for operating the camera is used to give image stability and optimal positioning.

Transperitoneal vs. extraperitoneal

The procedure may be transperitoneal with or without primary dissection of the seminal vesicles via the peritoneal reflection of the rectovesical pouch or it may be extraperitoneal using various means to develop the space anterior to the bladder. There are no specific anatomical contraindications for the transperitoneal approach although previous abdominal surgery can make this difficult, requiring time-consuming adhesiolysis. Extraperitoneal surgery can decrease operative time in this group as well as in obese patients. Previous laparoscopic mesh hernia repair is a relative contraindication for an extraperitoneal procedure due to difficulty in developing the space of Retzius. The main problem executing the extraperitoneal approach concerns the vesico-urethral anastomosis that is performed under more tension than the transperitoneal procedure. The tension stems from the fact that the bladder has not been completely mobilised as it has in transperitoneal prostatectomy. Levelling the table, emptying the bladder and freeing the bladder's attachments may resolve this. Anastomotic leakage is easier to manage after extraperitoneal surgery due to the absence of peritoneal irritation and ileus. Ureteric and bowel injury are less likely with extraperitoneal surgery although rectal injury risks are unchanged.

Surgical technique

Classically, LRP involves mobilisation of the prostate and bladder by excising the anterior fat and incising the endopelvic fascia bilaterally (Figure 9.2). The anterior dorsal venous complex is then ligated. The anterior and posterior bladder neck is divided,

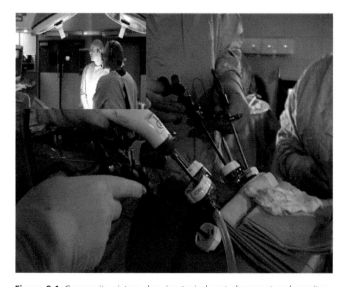

Figure 9.1 Composite picture showing typical port placement and monitor position.

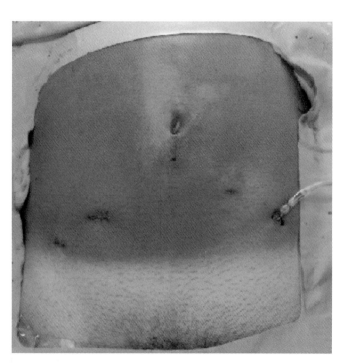

Figure 9.2 Typical immediate post-op appearance of abdomen.

dissection is continued posteriorly to deliver the seminal vesicals. The posterior leaf of Denonvillier's fascia is incised and the fatty plane between rectum and prostate developed. The lateral prostate pedicles are divided with release or excision of the neurovascular bundles. The decision-making process on how to deal with the neurovascular bundles starts pre-operatively with assessment of pre-operative erectile function and disease burden. This guides the balance between ensuring oncological control and preservation of erectile function. The distal apex of the prostate is then dissected and the urethra is divided. Haemostasis is secured and the posteriorly situated rectal wall is checked. In essence, the entire prostate is removed as well as the seminal vesicles. In addition, each vas is divided with the distal end being included in the surgical specimen. Men are therefore sterile following this procedure. The bladder is then brought down to the urethral stump and a circular anastamosis performed, either interrupted on continuous, around a urethral catheter. The catheter is removed at 7–10 days post-operatively.

Post-operative course

In general, patients recover well after LRP. Average post-operative hospital stay is one or two days. This is dependent upon pre-operative counselling including training patients in the use of a catheter, good post-operative analgesia and a surgical/nursing team focused on early mobilisation and discharge planning. However, . . .

Patients must not underestimate the degree of post-operative fatigue out of keeping with the small wounds. The surgical incisions are consistent with removal of small sebaceous cysts, however, this is major surgery. Common and not so common questions/problems/issues are listed below:

- Patients should not drive or cycle with a catheter.
- Heavy lifting is to be avoided for around six weeks.
- Patients should get back onto full diet only when they are passing flatus freely.
- Patients should not be straining at stool post-operatively. Lactulose is useful.

- Urine bypassing and peri-catheter blood and discharge are to be expected.
- If the catheter is blocked, the specialist team should be consulted. Changing a blocked catheter post radical prostatectomy can be disastrous if the new catheter disrupts the vesico-urethral anastamosis.

Complications – early

The commonest early post-op complications are urine leak and pelvic haematoma.

- Usually a urine leak is not an anastomotic disruption but a small hole siphoning preferentially down the drain.
- A pelvic haematoma usually presents as pain. The options are early exploration vs. prolonged catheterization if the diagnosis is delayed. This is necessary as the haematoma will cause a degree of anastomotic disruption.
- Urosepsis is the rarest complication following LRP. If a patient is septic, a bowel injury must be excluded with a soluble contrast enema with or without a contrast-enhanced CT. The only definitive test to identify a low rectal injury is a gastrograffin enema.
- Port hernias are rare.
- Similar incidence is reported for late inguinal hernias in the age-matched population.

Complications – late

- Persistent incontinence – If a patient is wet, accept it and refer for a specialist continence opinion. Only then can the patient decide to put up with it, wait and see or decide on a surgical solution.
- Erectile dysfunction – If a patient has significant erectile dysfunction and is bothered, address it. Refer them to the erectile dysfunction team. There should be someone with a special interest in this group. There will be a solution with tablets, pellets, pumps, injections, bands or prosthesis.

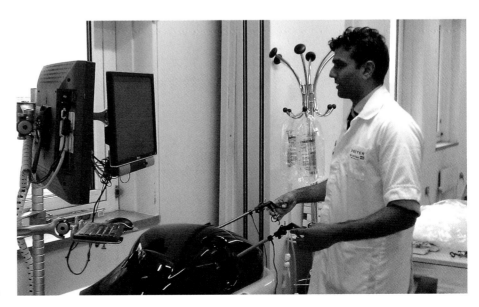

Figure 9.3 Typical dry lab 'training box' in use.

Table 9.1 Comparative costs of prostatectomy.

Financial summary	Open (£)	Laparoscopic (£)	Robotic (£)
National tariff	4974	4736	4974
Less 30% for Trust overheads	3482	3315	3482
Robotic surgery top-up tariff			2601
Consumables	−605	−750	−2500
Consultant cost	−250	−200	−250
Junior cost	0	0	0
Theatre cost	−1740	−1392	−1740
Ward stay	−1003	−453	−678
Robot servicing and maintenance			−675
Theatre time extension			−700
Sub-total	−116	520	240
Two cases per day	−232	1040	480
Theatre time extension			−700
Total	−232	1040	−220
at 200 per year	−23200	104000	−22000

Training

LRP is most likely delivered by a dedicated surgeon, willing to invest time and energy in continuous learning and improvement, in a high volume centre with a continuous audit of outcome to indicate the need for improvement. It is important to be able to disseminate the technique safely and effectively. That is to say, one must be able to teach the technique so that it can be taken up with minimal negative outcomes during the learning curve. LRP involves a difficult and complex combination of skills to be able to control the instruments effectively, which requires a great deal of exacting practice and a multitude of surgical steps that need to be performed perfectly to achieve the target goals. The latter requires a detailed knowledge of the operation from open surgical experience or fellowship training and an attitude to strive for perfection by reflecting on every step in detail and striving to improve. Thus, 80 hours of dry lab suturing (Figure 9.3), 80 cases as an assistant and 80 cases as primary surgeon are not unrealistic goals of training.

Cost

Being able to deliver a cost-effective radical prostatectomy within the financial constraints of the healthcare system is important although secondary to oncological, functional and safety outcomes, which are, however, more a reflection of surgeon technique and volume. The comparative costs at the authors' institution where all the techniques are practised are demonstrated in Table 9.1. LRP is the most cost-effective method despite the top-up tariff for robotic surgery.

Conclusion

Broadly, there is good evidence that radical prostatectomy may be performed well by whichever means is chosen. Dedicated surgeons in high volume, well-supported institutions produce better results than those in low-volume programmes. Patients should choose their surgeon and hospital before their technique. Laparoscopic surgery has clear theoretical advantages over open surgery if both are compared when performed expertly. For patient, surgeon and managers, this holds true. The technical difficulty, the very long learning curve and the difficulty training surgeons in this technique limit its dissemination in the era of robotic surgery. Learning curves should belong to high volume institutions not individuals. Mentoring within high volume institutions will limit the morbidity of learning curves for patients.

Further reading

Guillonneau B, Vallancien G. Laparoscopic radical prostatectomy: The Montsouris technique. *J Urol* 2000;**163**(6):1643–9.

Rassweiler J, Seemann O, Schulze M, Teber D, Hatzinger M, Frede T. Laparoscopic versus open radical prostatectomy: a comparative study at a single institution. *J Urol* 2003;**169**(5):1689–93.

Vickers AJ, Savage CJ, Hruza M, Tuerk I, Koenig P, Martínez-Piñeiro L, Janetschek G, Guillonneau B. The surgical learning curve for laparoscopic radical prostatectomy: a retrospective cohort study. *Lancet Oncology* 2009;**10**(5):475–80.

CHAPTER 10

Robotic Radical Prostatectomy

Ben Challacombe[1] and Jim Peabody[2]

[1]Guy's and St. Thomas' Hospital NHS Foundation Trust, London, UK
[2]Henry Ford Hospital, Detroit, MI, USA

OVERVIEW

- Introduction to robotic prostatectomy and its history
- Robotic technology
- Surgical approach and techniques
- Outcomes
- Controversies

Introduction

Urologists have been at the forefront of the current drive towards minimally invasive surgical treatments especially with regards to localised prostate cancer. It soon became obvious in the late 1990s that laparoscopic radical prostatectomy (LRP) was an extremely difficult technique with a long learning curve that many urological surgeons were failing to overcome. The operation was often very long, required complex skills, and placed significant mental and physical strain on the surgeon, particularly during suturing. When a French team came to teach LRP to a group of US surgeons at the Henry Ford Centre in Detroit, a new robotic system was being trialled and the collaborative group switched over to the new system with almost immediate success. Robotic-assisted radical prostatectomy (RARP) is considered by many to be the new gold standard approach to radical prostatectomy and has come a long way since the first procedure by Claude Abbou in Créteil, France, in 2001. The launch of the da Vinci® master-slave robotic system (Figure 10.1), named after Leonardo da Vinci's robotic knight, by Intuitive Surgical, in 2001 provided a platform for minimally invasive prostatectomy that was more straightforward to learn and easier for open surgeons to transfer to than laparoscopic prostatectomy.

As a result, over 1000 of these da Vinci systems have been acquired in the United States where over 70% of radical prostatectomies are now performed robotically along with many other urological procedures and operations in other surgical disciplines. The UK currently has 27 systems, with several more planned. There are several other surgical robots in clinical use such as the

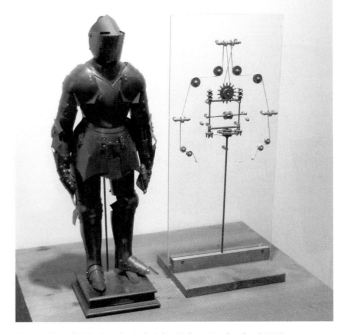

Figure 10.1 da Vinci's robotic knight. (Release Under the GNU Free Document Licence).

older Zeus™ master slave system and the ASEOP robot, a robotic camera/instrument holder, but none have penetrated the surgical marketplace with anything like the success of the da Vinci.

Robotic technology

The da Vinci robot is the primary operative robot throughout the world and was originally conceived as a means of remotely operating in space or on the battlefield. It is not a true 'robot' but rather a master-slave system consisting of three major parts; the operating console that is non-sterile and placed separately to the patient, the endoscopic stack containing the light source and insufflation equipment, and the surgical cart itself with three or usually four robotic arms (Figures 10.2 and 10.3).

The initial standard system has been upgraded to a da Vinci S, Si, or S HD. The system uses stereoscopic viewing with dual cameras (Figure 10.4) to immerse the surgeon in a three-dimensional

ABC of Prostate Cancer, First Edition.
Edited by Prokar Dasgupta and Roger S. Kirby.
© 2012 Blackwell Publishing Ltd. Published 2012 by Blackwell Publishing Ltd.

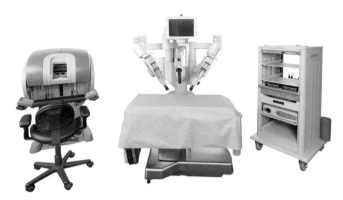

Figure 10.2 da Vinci console, cart and stack. Courtesy of Intuitive Surgical: from the Intuitive Surgical Website.

operating field. The surgeon's console contains the master controls that the surgeon uses to manipulate the instruments. The surgeon's forefinger and thumb sit on the handles or 'Masters' which intuitively translate the surgeon's natural hand and wrist movements into corresponding, precise and scaled movements of the robotic arms (Figure 10.5). This extensive range of motion allows precision that is not available in standard laparoscopic procedures. These 'Endowrist™' instruments have six degrees of freedom and are only able to move when commanded by the surgeon (Figures 10.4 and 10.6).

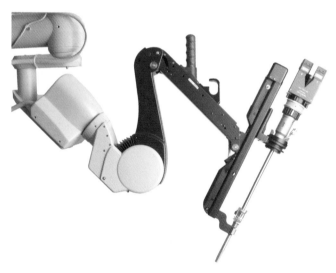

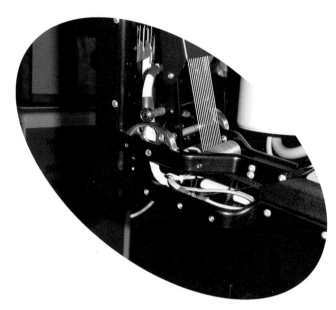

Figure 10.5 da Vinci arm mechanism. Courtesy of Intuitive Surgical: from the Intuitive Surgical Website.

Figure 10.3 da Vinci S robotic arm. Courtesy of Intuitive Surgical: from the Intuitive Surgical Website.

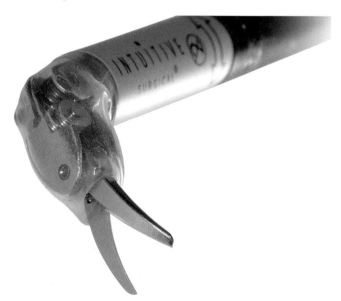

Figure 10.4 da Vinci Endowrist scissors. Courtesy of Intuitive Surgical: from the Intuitive Surgical Website.

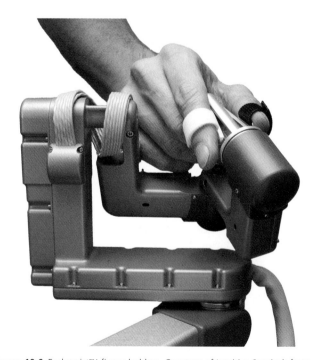

Figure 10.6 Endowrist™ finger holders. Courtesy of Intuitive Surgical: from the Intuitive Surgical Website.

There is almost complete removal of tremor and there is also motion scaling of the instruments by a factor of 3, 5 or 10:1. The primary surgeon is comfortably seated at the console providing ergonomic positioning and allowing the operation to occur in comfort. It is even possible to have the surgeon positioned some distance from the patient outside the main operating room (Figures 10.7 and 10.8).

The usual benefits of minimally invasive surgery are reported by most centres performing RARP, including reduced blood loss and the need for blood transfusion, reduced post-operative pain, reduced scarring, an earlier hospital discharge in most centres and an earlier return to work or normal activity. There are also potential benefits in terms of improved cancer control by reducing positive surgical margins, earlier return to full continence and improved identification and preservation of the cavernous nerves for erectile function. The latter do not have level I evidence.

The da Vinci robotic system is generally most useful in procedures which have a reconstructive element requiring the surgeon to cut

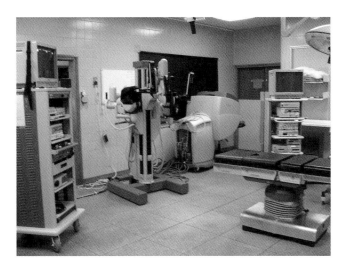

Figure 10.7 Robotic theatre set-up.

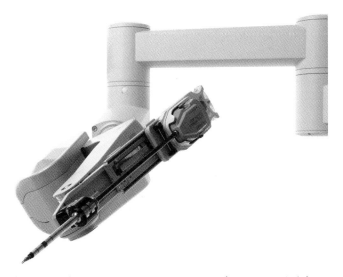

Figure 10.8 da Vinci S instrument arm. Courtesy of Intuitive Surgical: from the Intuitive Surgical Website.

and suture at awkward angles. Dry lab training can improve surgical skills in this area. It is also possible that the improved dexterity and visualisation may allow a more precise procedure with fewer complications.

Surgical approach and technique

Approach

Most centres use a trans-peritoneal approach but an extra-peritoneal technique is also possible. The patient is placed supine with Trendelenberg tilt (head down) following securing to prevent operative sliding. A urethral catheter is placed and the pneumoperitoneum is established using either a Verres needle or the open Hassan technique. Six robotic/laparoscopic ports are introduced and the robot is docked onto the patient. Most centres employ an anterograde dissection to the prostate from the bladder neck forward to the prostatic apex.

Mobilisation and dorsal venous complex control

Any obstructing intra-peritoneal adhesions are taken down and the small bowel/sigmoid colon pushed cranially to make space. The bladder is mobilised from the anterior abdominal wall, dropped down, the endopelvic fascia incised and peri-prostatic fat cleared. The dorsal vascular complex to the prostate is identified and generally sutured with one or two interrupted dissolvable sutures. The complex may be suspended from the pubis anteriorly to aid haemostasis and assist continence.

Bladder neck, seminal vesicles/vasa, and posterior dissection

The anterior bladder neck is divided close to the prostate and the ureteric orifices identified and avoided. The posterior bladder neck is divided, Denonvillier's fascia is incised and the seminal vesicles and vasa are identified and mobilised using as little thermal energy as possible.

Pedicle control and nerve sparing

The vascular pedicles to the prostate are divided using Hem-o-Lok clips or metal ligaclips. Occasionally if nerve-sparing is not required, e.g. in locally advanced disease or when operating on an impotent patient, diathermy is used. Generally an athermal technique is used to peel the neurovascular bundles away from the prostate towards the apex of the gland. Pre-operative assessment including the numbers of positive biopsies, the Gleason grade, MRI findings and clinical stage will determine the degree of erectile nerve preservation that is attempted for each side.

Apical dissection and reconstruction

The apex of the prostate is dissected and the urethra is divided. The specimen is placed into an endoscopic bag for later retrieval. A running anastomosis using monofilament suture is performed with 10–12 bites on each side and a knot is tied anteriorly (Figure 10.9). A large two-way urethral catheter is inserted and the anastomosis leak tested to ensure its integrity.

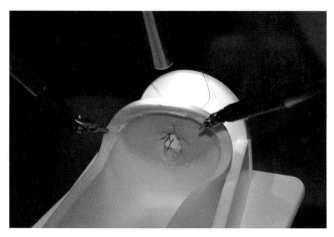

Figure 10.9 Vesico-urethral anastomosis model. Courtesy of Mr Declan Murphy.

Closure, drain, management

A drain is placed through a port site with its end near the anastomosis, the specimen is retrieved from the peri-umbilical port and the individual ports are closed with deeper fascial sutures for the larger ones. The patient can move after 2–4 hours, and the drain is removed the next morning if dry. A soft diet is maintained until the bowels open normally and the patient can usually go home on post-operative day 1 or 2. The catheter is removed at 7–14 days depending on the centre and a cystogram may be performed to check for anastomotic leakage prior to catheter removal.

Outcomes data

In order to be successful, RARP needed to match the oncological and functional outcomes of open radical prostatectomy while providing the additional benefits of the minimally invasive approach. The fact that so few surgeons have gone back to the open approach having experienced RARP is testament to its ability to achieve these goals. Patients are rarely transfused, may go home after 24 hours, have low complication rates (Clavien Grade $\geq$3 circa 5%). The overall success of radical prostatectomy by any technique is measured by the so-called 'trifecta' of oncological control, urinary continence and erectile function. Several very high-volume centres have published outcomes that are comparable to the best in the history of open surgery. It has become increasingly clear that the individual surgeon's skill and experience are extremely important to clinical outcomes whichever surgical approach is employed. With this in mind, the positive margin rates for RARP are encouraging with rates for T2 and T3 disease at around 10–15% and 30–40% in most published series with some centres quoting rates as low as 5 and 25% respectively. Long-term oncological data are still awaited in most centres due to the novelty of the technique and the relative immaturity of the follow-up, however, early signs are very encouraging.

Regarding functional outcome data, this is a difficult area to assess due to the initial lack of standardisation of terminology between some centres. Generally most units would expect a continence rate at one year post RARP of over 90% as defined by no pad use or a single security pad. With regards erectile dysfunction in men undergoing RARP who have had a full bilateral nerve spare, most quote rates of penetrative intercourse of between 50–70% depending on the patients' age and pre-existing erectile function.

Controversies

The major controversies regarding RARP surround the marketing of the robotic system itself and the reporting of oncological and functional outcome measures. There is little doubt that the introduction of RARP has served to raise the bar for all approaches to radical prostatectomy, both in terms of how specific outcomes are recorded and the measures of quality expected by the surgeons and patients alike. The excellent vision afforded by the da Vinci system has allowed urological surgeons to appreciate anatomy that was previously very difficult to accurately see. The focus on the technical nuances of the procedure has been immense. However, RARP is certainly not easy to learn and requires significant dedication and practice, but it is easier to grasp and perfect than LRP. This has opened the field of minimally invasive prostate cancer surgery to a larger number of surgeons, many of whom have little or no previous laparoscopic experience but can now produce excellent results.

It is also true that many of the 'benefits' of RARP are excessively marketed by industry and individual robotic surgeons. Most major centres report outstanding oncological and functional outcomes when compared to the historical series of open radical prostatectomy. The drive towards further innovation in this area is huge with talk of new robotic platforms, intra-operative imaging and tissue analysis. There are no large RCTs in this area and as patients become increasingly well informed, the window of opportunity for trials to occur may already have passed. For the patient, the benefits of minimally invasive surgery are compelling and RARP is certainly here to stay. It looks to be the current gold standard for radical prostatectomy.

Further reading

Ficarra V, Novara G, Artibani W, Cestari A, Galfano A, Graefen M, et al. Retropubic, laparoscopic, and robot-assisted radical prostatectomy: A systematic review and cumulative analysis of comparative studies. *Eur Urol* 2009;**55**:1037–63.

Murphy DG, Bjartell A, Ficarra V, Graefen M, Haese A, Montironi R, et al. Downsides of robot-assisted laparoscopic radical prostatectomy: Limitations and complications. *Eur Urol* 2010; **57**:735–46.

Patel, VR (ed.). *Robotic Urologic Surgery* 2nd edn. Berlin: Springer Publishers, 2010.

Patel VR, Palmer KJ, Coughlin G, Samavedi S. Robotic-assisted laparoscopic radical prostatectomy: Perioperative outcomes of 1500 cases. *J Endourol* 2008;**22**:2299–306.

Smith J, Tewari A. *Robotics in Urologic Surgery*. Oxford: Elsevier Publishers, 2008.

CHAPTER 11

Prostate Brachytherapy

Peter Acher and Rick Popert

Department of Urology, Guy's and St Thomas' Hospital NHS Foundation Trust, London, UK

OVERVIEW

- Prostate brachytherapy is a form of targeted radiotherapy
- Brachytherapy offers a day-case radical treatment option for localised prostate cancer with a favourable morbidity profile
- Data beyond 12 years demonstrate the efficacy of prostate brachytherapy
- Modern techniques allow patients with large prostates or prior transurethral resection of the prostate to be treated
- Brachytherapy may be combined with external beam radiotherapy for higher risk patients, and may be used as a salvage treatment option after failed radiotherapy

Introduction

Brachytherapy is a form of radiotherapy. Rather than apply the energy in the form of X-rays from outside the body as in external beam radiotherapy (EBRT), radioactive sources that emit gamma rays are placed directly in, or in close proximity to the prostate gland. Data from several longitudinal studies inform us that oncological control is directly dependent on prescribed dose. Doses from EBRT, however, are limited by toxicity to the surrounding organs at risk (bladder, urethra and rectum) – also related to dose. The inverse square law governs the dose from a brachytherapy source such that there is a rapid fall-off of dose a short distance from the origin. Multiple sources, each with a 'cloud' of radiation, can be placed in such a configuration so as to provide a high dose to the prostate whilst minimising dose, and toxicity, to the surrounding structures.

Prostate brachytherapy sources may be permanent in the form of seeds, or temporary (also known as high dose rate) with iridium wires. Temporary prostate brachytherapy is currently considered developmental. The seeds used in permanent low dose rate implants consist of titanium capsules, 4.5 by 0.8 mm, which encapsulate the radioactive sources. Palladium-123, Caesium-131 and Iodine-125 isotopes are all used although none have been shown to be superior in terms of either toxicity or disease control. For practical

purposes, Iodine-125 is used in the UK. Iodine-125 has a half-life of approximately 60 days and so an implant is considered active for ten months, or five half-lives. A typical Iodine-125 implant with a prescribed dose of 145 Gy will deliver the biological equivalent of up to 90 Gy of EBRT. Approximately 70 sources are used for a 40 cm^3 gland.

Technique development

The development of trans-rectal ultrasound in the early 1980s allowed accurate placement of brachytherapy sources via the trans-perineal route under image guidance. The early technique was developed in Seattle as a two-stage procedure. At first, the patient is placed in a lithotomy position and images of the prostate, urethra and rectum are captured. Those images are then used to plan the implant in relation to a brachytherapy grid placed over the perineum. At a later date, the patient returns for the implant: under anaesthetic the patient's position is replicated as accurately as possible to match the pre-plan study; the sources, usually on strands, are placed according to the plan using preloaded needles inserted through the grid (Figure 11.1). A post-operative CT scan is commonly utilised in order to detect the seed positions in relation to the prostate and assess the dosimetry.

The technique has evolved to a single-stage procedure with the use of nomograms and subsequent computerised planning systems that avoid issues with reproducing the pre-plan position. An inverse technique refers to the placement of needles before planning so that difficulties in reaching areas of the prostate (such as behind the pubic arch) can be overcome by adjusting the position intraoperatively. Sources are placed individually in an 'after-loaded' manner. Modern techniques, known as dynamic dose-feedback, not only use computer software to create the inverse plan intraoperatively, but also record each seed position as it is placed in real time, and update the dosimetry accordingly (Figures 11.2 and 11.3). This allows on-table adjustments to be made before the patient leaves the operating room.

Side effects

The treatment is usually carried out as a day-case procedure and patients report a rapid return to usual daily activity. The implant is radioactive and bearing this in mind, men are asked to avoid

ABC of Prostate Cancer, First Edition.
Edited by Prokar Dasgupta and Roger S. Kirby.
© 2012 Blackwell Publishing Ltd. Published 2012 by Blackwell Publishing Ltd.

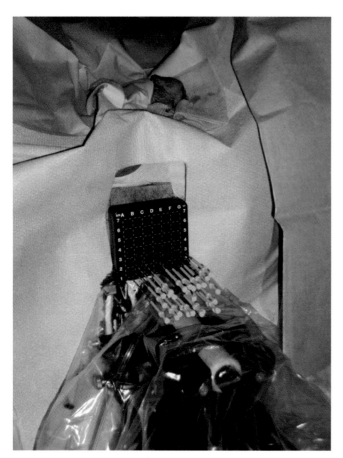

Figure 11.1 Needles are placed transperineally through a brachytherapy grid, parallel to a trans-rectal ultrasound probe and under image guidance. Aerosolized gel helps visualize the urethra. The patient is in an extended lithotomy position.

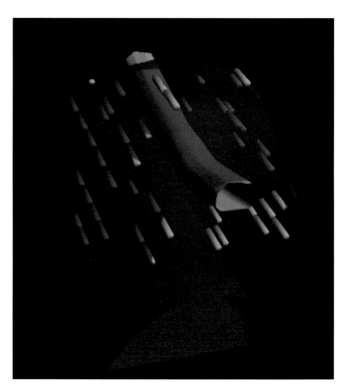

Figure 11.2 Three-dimensional representation of implant. The prostate is in red, urethra, green, and rectum, blue. The discrete green cylinders are radioactive seeds.

prolonged contact with pregnant women and small children for a period of two months. Similarly, seeds may be emitted in the semen with ejaculation and so a condom is recommended for the first three emissions.

A degree of urinary symptoms occur in the majority of men: initially there may be a reduction of flow due to swelling of the gland during the procedure. Retention rates are low (approximately 5%) and usually recover after a short period of catheterisation. In men who require catheterisation for longer (1%), definitive therapy (such as transurethral resection) should be delayed for a year in order to allow the implant to treat the cancer and for resolution of radiation-associated symptoms. During this time, men may be managed with either intermittent self-catheterisation or a supra-pubic catheter.

Radiation effects cause irritative urinary symptoms that peak at four to six weeks, but usually settle to baseline by nine months (Figure 11.4). Alpha-blockers are routinely prescribed and anti-cholinergics along with fluid advice are often helpful. Radiation effects on the bowel may cause diarrhoea in 5% of men and, rarely, bleeding occurs; this is self-limiting. Erectile function is commonly preserved following brachytherapy implant, at least for the first few years, with or without the use of phosphodiesterase-5 inhibitors.

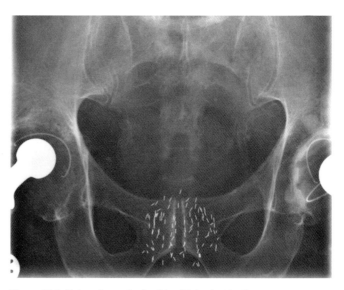

Figure 11.3 Plain radiograph of pelvis with implant in situ.

Cancer control

Oncological surveillance is managed by serial PSA measurements. As with EBRT, the PSA can take up to two years and sometimes longer to fall to its nadir level. One-third of patients experience a 'PSA bounce', whereby the PSA rises before falling again towards its nadir. The dosimetry review, either by post-operative CT images or on-table dynamic assessment, will ensure satisfactory coverage. The D90 refers to the minimum dose that 90% of the prostate receives;

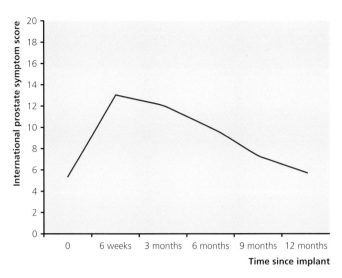

Figure 11.4 Urinary symptoms following prostate brachytherapy implant: mean international prostate symptom scores.

Table 11.1 Comparison of radical treatments for localised prostate cancer.

	External beam radiotherapy	Radical prostatectomy	Brachytherapy
Anaesthesia	Nil	Required	Required
Hospital stay	Treatment visits daily for 6 weeks	1–7 nights	Day-case procedure
Catheterisation	Uncommon	7–10 days	5% 1 week 1% require delayed surgery
Urinary symptoms	Irritative	Incontinence, 50% early 5% long term	Irritative
Erectile dysfunction	Secondary to hormones	Common	Uncommon. May occur several years later.
Rectal symptoms	30%	Rare rectal injury	5%
Time to daily activities	6 weeks	4–8 weeks	<1 week

a D90 of more than 130Gy has been associated with improved outcomes. Data up to 12 years have shown biochemical control in the order of 90% of patients with low risk disease. A cohort study concerning men with T1 to T2 disease treated without hormones, compared radical prostatectomy (n = 746), EBRT to a median dose of 74 Gy (n = 340) and permanent prostate brachytherapy (n = 733) demonstrated similar seven-year freedom from biochemical recurrence results of 74–79% (statistically insignificant differences).

Patient assessment

As with any treatment for prostate cancer, patient selection is important. NICE guidelines recommend prostate brachytherapy for low and intermediate risk localised disease. Higher risk patients may be treated with a combination of brachytherapy and EBRT: this allows maximum dose to the prostate as well as treatment doses to a margin (in case of extracapsular extension) while still protecting surrounding tissues. Transperineal sector prostate biopsies are particularly useful for disease stratification when planning treatment options. Since the patient position is similar to that of the implant, the accessibility of the gland can be ascertained. The co-ordinates of higher grade or volume of disease can be recorded and these areas targeted with extra dose during the implant procedure.

Urinary symptom score and uroflowmetry are important aspects of pre-brachytherapy assessment. High symptom scores and poor flow are predictors of urinary morbidity following the implant. Patients with equivocal flow rates ought to undergo further urodynamic evaluation. Men with low-risk and low-volume disease who would otherwise be suitable for active surveillance but who have bladder outflow obstruction secondary to prostatic disease may be managed by transurethral resection of the prostate followed by implant six months later. The surgery is best carried out by a urologist familiar with brachytherapy implants.

In the past, large prostate sizes were considered a relative contraindication to brachytherapy implant due to the increased urinary symptoms following the procedure and difficulties with access to the anterior part of the gland (Figure 11.4). Downsizing has been achieved with LHRH analogues prior to implant, but with associated morbidity. Inverse plan techniques overcome pubic arch interference, however, and providing there are no signs of bladder outflow obstruction, prostate glands larger than 50 cm³ may be implanted with satisfactory dosimetric and urinary outcomes.

Similarly, patients with prior bladder outflow surgery were previously considered poor candidates for implant due to historical data reporting incontinence in these men and difficulties in achieving dose coverage. Modern techniques and equipment, however, allow more targeted placement of seeds so that a history of transurethral resection of the prostate need not be a contraindication, providing there is an adequate rim of prostate tissue to implant.

More recently, the indications for brachytherapy have extended to its use as a salvage treatment for radiotherapy failure with promising results. As our understanding of radiation biology evolves and imaging and targeting of dose continue to improve, the indications for and results of this treatment will likely expand. At present, prostate brachytherapy offers a radical treatment option with relatively low morbidity and the convenience of a day-case procedure. Table 11.1 presents a comparison of radical treatments for localised prostate cancer.

Further reading

National Institute for Health and Clinical Excellence. *Prostate Cancer: Diagnosis and Treatment*. London: NICE, 2008 (www.nice.org.uk/CG058).

Potters L, Calugaru E, Jassal A, Presser J. Is there a role for postimplant dosimetry after real-time dynamic permanent prostate brachytherapy? *Int J Radiat Oncol Biol Phys* 2006;**65**(4):1014–19.

Potters L, Klein EA, Kattan MW, Reddy CA, Ciezki JP, Reuther AM, Kupelian PA. Monotherapy for stage T1-T2 prostate cancer: Radical prostatectomy, external beam radiotherapy, or permanent seed implantation. *Radiother Oncol* 2004;**71**(1):29–33.

Prostate Brachytherapy Advisory Group UK and Ireland. (www.prostatebrachytherapyinfo.net).

Stock RG, Stone NN, Cesaretti JA, Rosenstein BS. Biologically effective dose values for prostate brachytherapy: Effects on PSA failure and posttreatment biopsy results. *Int J Radiat Oncol Biol Phys* 2006;**64**(2):527–33.

CHAPTER 12

HIFU

Louise Dickinson[1], Hashim U. Ahmed[1] and Mark Emberton[2]

[1]Division of Surgery and Interventional Sciences, University College Hospital London, London, UK
[2]University College Hospital London, London, UK

OVERVIEW

- High intensity focused ultrasound (HIFU) is a relatively new treatment for prostate cancer that uses focused ultrasound waves to heat tissue and cause localised necrosis of tissue

- HIFU is currently used to treat the whole prostate in men with localised prostate cancer as an alternative to other therapies such as radiotherapy or other types of surgery (e.g. prostatectomy)

- The two HIFU devices in clinical practice are the Ablatherm® (EDAP-TMS SA, Vaulx en Velin, France) and Sonablate 500® (Focus Surgery Inc, Indianapolis, IN)

- Cancer-free outcomes for primary whole gland treatment are approximately 90% from recent published data. Cancer outcomes and side effect profiles are poorer in salvage HIFU cases

- Treating only the areas of cancer in the prostate with focal HIFU may become an important new therapy that treats the cancer effectively but with fewer side effects. This is an area that is currently being explored within the clinical trial setting

Introduction

Management of prostate cancer has been evolving towards an era of minimal access in order to reduce the significant over-treatment burden of traditional radical therapies. Despite refinements in surgery (robot-assisted and laparoscopic prostatectomy) and radiotherapy (intensity modulation), the beneficial impact on functional outcomes has been less than certain. High intensity focused ultrasound (HIFU), a minimally invasive therapy that can be delivered in an ambulatory care setting, is repeatable, and may have the potential to reduce the morbidity of therapy while maintaining acceptable cancer control.

History of HIFU

HIFU uses ultrasound waves that, when targeted to small areas, are capable of heating tissue to over 60°C, causing irreversible tissue

ABC of Prostate Cancer, First Edition.
Edited by Prokar Dasgupta and Roger S. Kirby.
© 2012 Blackwell Publishing Ltd. Published 2012 by Blackwell Publishing Ltd.

destruction. Its therapeutic application was first described in 1942 by Lynn et al. when neurological changes were noted in cats and dogs in which brain tissue was treated. However, it was not until the 1950s that its application was targeted on cancer tissue, with clinical evaluation on both benign and malignant prostate tissue starting to be of interest in the 1990s. Although HIFU has not been proven to be a successful alternative treatment of benign prostatic hyperplasia to TURP (transurethral resection of the prostate), it is its ability to ablate tumours with an acceptable side-effect profile that has resulted in its adoption as a form of cancer therapy worldwide.

As well as within the prostate, HIFU therapy has been applied to a number of other fields, including liver, bladder, kidney and breast cancers, as well as brain tissue for patients with Parkinson's disease, and in the uterus for ablation of fibroids. However, all of these treatments are at different stages of clinical development, with most undergoing evaluation of medium- to long-term outcomes within ongoing clinical trials.

Physical principles of HIFU

HIFU uses the mechanisms of thermal ablation and cavitation to cause irreversible cell damage. High frequency vibrations originating from a transducer produce ultrasound waves. These are focused on a target area (approximately 10 mm long and 2 mm wide), depositing large amounts of energy, which is absorbed by the tissue and converted into heat. Temperatures up to 100°C can be reached for a period of a few seconds, causing necrosis and cell death within the target area without causing damage to the surrounding tissue.

Cavitation can also occur as a result of interaction between the ultrasound and micro-bubbles within treated tissue.

Platforms and procedure

There are currently two HIFU devices available for the treatment of prostate cancer: the Ablatherm® (EDAP-TMS SA, Vaulx en Velin, France) and the Sonablate 500® (Focus Surgery Inc, Indianapolis, IN) (Figure 12.1). There are differences in technology and conduct between them. However, both involve the delivery of treatment via a trans-rectal probe containing the transducer. Treatment effects can be monitored via real-time ultrasound. In most cases, the patient receives a general anaesthetic. This allows for patient tolerance and restricts motion so that accurate targeting is possible. The rectum is

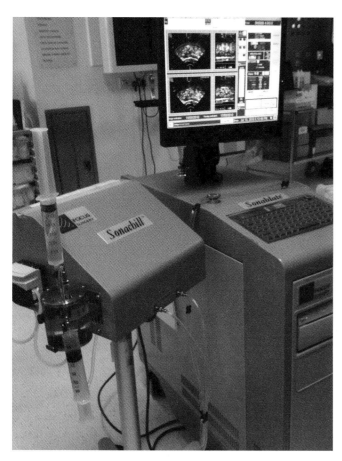

Figure 12.1 The Sonablate® 500 HIFU device.

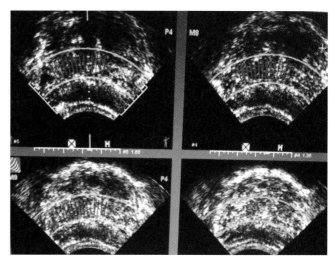

Figure 12.2 HIFU treatment planning: the surgeon places bars within a treatment zone, in the areas he wishes to treat.

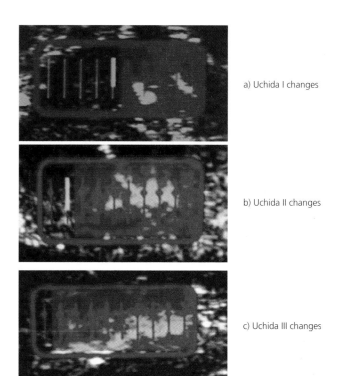

a) Uchida I changes

b) Uchida II changes

c) Uchida III changes

Figure 12.3 Uchida changes are represented as: (a) grade I – discrete rather than confluent grey-scale changes within the treatment zone; (b) grade II – confluent change within the treatment zone; and (c) grade III – greyscale changes migrating outside the treatment zone; grade III represents 'over-treatment'.

cooled during treatment using continuous irrigation with degassed water in order to limit the potential adverse effects of heating, e.g. fistula formation.

The Ablatherm® device consists of two 'modules': the treatment module on which the patient lies in a lateral position to receive treatment, and the control module where the surgeon plans treatment and controls the position of the probe delivering HIFU. Treatment plans are automated to a pre-set protocol depending on whether it is a primary treatment, re-treatment, or salvage procedure (cancer recurrence following a previous form of radical treatment). The Sonablate 500® equipment consists of a monitoring module together with the transrectal probe which is inserted with the patient supine and in the lithotomy position on a standard operating table. The Sonablate 500® is controlled manually by the surgeon and the power of HIFU pulses can be altered according to real-time visual feedback from the ultrasound images (Figure 12.2).

Currently, ultrasound is the modality by which real-time feedback of treatment effects is received. These can be seen as greyscale changes as the heating effect causes tissue damage. However, MRI is currently being evaluated for this purpose, both for prostate cancer and other forms of disease treated with HIFU. MRI-guided HIFU may provide a more precise localisation of the cancer for treatment planning, and provide information on tissue temperature changes to limit the risk of inadequate cancer control (under-heating) versus increased side effect risks from over-heating. The power

delivered can be altered immediately by the surgeon according to the real-time effects seen. At present, MR-guided HIFU is being evaluated as part of clinical trials.

Thermal effects of treatment on ultrasound can be seen as grey-scale changes, so-called 'Uchida changes'. These changes have been classified into grades of I, II and III depending on the extent of the greyscale changes within the targeted area (Figure 12.3).

Indications

Although short- and medium-term data for oncological and functional outcomes are promising, longer-term outcomes of atleast 10 years are currently not known. Patients should be made aware of this prior to committing to a management preference.

HIFU is considered an alternative primary treatment option to other forms of radical therapy (e.g. radical prostatectomy, radiotherapy, brachytherapy) for men with low–intermediate risk localised prostate cancer (T1-T2cN0M0, PSA ≤ 15, Gleason < 7). In some centres, patients with radiological T3a disease are also considered, but this option should be limited to practitioners with sufficient experience.

Further prostate treatment is not precluded if cancer recurrence occurs. Patients can either undergo further HIFU or be considered for brachytherapy, cryotherapy, radiotherapy or surgery. The majority of men choose to have redo HIFU so the numbers undergoing other therapeutic modalities is low. Therefore, the toxicity profile of radical therapies after HIFU is poorly reported but would be expected to be higher than if these were applied to a naïve gland. HIFU can also be offered as a salvage procedure when other forms of treatment, usually radiotherapy, have failed in men with non-metastatic recurrence. It may offer definitive cancer control or a delayed requirement for palliative hormone ablation therapy in this sub-group.

Contra-indications

Prostate-related contra-indications to HIFU treatment include a large prostate size, whereby the focal length for treatment would not reach the anterior part of the prostate. Some surgeons perform a TURP prior to HIFU to reduce the prostatic volume. Also, large calcium deposits within the prostate can prevent ultrasound wave propagation, causing under-treatment. Both of these factors can be assessed at a pre-operative trans-rectal ultrasound of the prostate. Non-prostatic reasons for HIFU exclusion include any anatomical or pathological abnormality limiting insertion of the rectal probe, e.g. tight anal stenosis, previous ano-rectal surgery.

Summary of published results

Primary HIFU

The first report of prostate cancer HIFU in humans was published in 1995 by Madersbacher et al. Local cancer control was poor in the early stages (approximately 50% of patients) but is continuing to improve as the technology is better understood and clinical experience is advancing.

PSA surveillance for monitoring disease recurrence is the norm following radical radiotherapy or prostatectomy. However, the ability of serial PSA results to detect recurrence following HIFU is less clear. Criteria that have been used to determine cancer-free status following HIFU include the ASTRO criteria, i.e. three consecutive rises in PSA following a PSA nadir, or the ASTRO-Phoenix criteria (nadir plus 2 ng/ml). Biochemical-free survival using these ASTRO criteria was reported as 75% by a group in Japan (Uchida et al. 2006) in 2006. More recently, rates of 85–92% are being achieved,

Table 12.1 Typical side effect profiles for primary whole prostate HIFU.

	Rate (%)
Symptomatic urinary tract infection	5
Urethral stricture	10–40
Retrograde ejaculation	3
Epididymitis	3
Urinary retention requiring surgery	2
Impotence	25–30
Incontinence (transient)	0–2
Recto-urethral fistula	<0.5

including within the first published primary whole gland HIFU trial in the UK in 2009 (Ahmed et al. 2009), although follow-up is short.

The main side effects and their published rates are detailed in Table 12.1.

Salvage HIFU

Patients undergoing any form of salvage therapy have a higher risk of side effects and diminished functional outcomes, and are therefore a difficult group of patients to treat. Recurrence rates following radiotherapy are approximately 30%. The side effects reported in a UK series of men undergoing whole gland HIFU for locally recurrent disease following radiotherapy (Zacharakis et al.) included stricture or intervention to remove necrotic tissue (36%), urinary tract infection or dysuria (26%), urinary incontinence (7%) and recto-urethral fistula (3%). Cancer control was achieved in 71% but median follow-up was limited to less than a year. These results are consistent with other published data. Murat et al. (2009) showed a local cancer control of 73% following salvage HIFU in 167 patients. However, those men with worsening cancer stage prior to EBRT, an increase in PSA prior to HIFU, or the use of hormone ablation therapy at any stage of their prostate cancer treatment had poorer disease-free outcomes. Careful patient selection is critically important to ensure that the risks of the treatment do not potentially outweigh the benefits of cancer control. The key issue is that up to 50% of men who have failed radiotherapy have micro-metastatic disease that is not detectable on current imaging modalities (MRI, bone scan, or PET).

Future applications

The ability of HIFU to ablate small discrete areas of tissue within millimetres of precision has led to an interest in its clinical application as a focal therapy. If cancerous tissue can be successfully and definitively ablated while preserving normal tissue, this potentially offers men a cancer treatment that minimises the functional impact as adjacent structures such as neurovascular bundles, external urinary sphincter, bladder neck and rectum, are avoided. Accurate localisation of cancer is required to ensure careful and appropriate patient selection, and this may be best performed with trans-perineal template prostate biopsies, where biopsies taken at 5 mm intervals, using a grid, provide an accurate 'mapping' of the prostate. Imaging is likely to have an important role with multi-parametric MRI, which uses several types of MRI, including

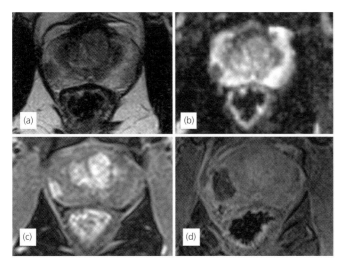

Figure 12.4 Focal HIFU for localised prostate cancer. The cancer is shown in the right posterior peripheral zone on the individual sequences of the multi-parametric MRI. (a) T2-weighted MRI; (b) diffusion-weighted MRI; (c) dynamic contrast enhanced MRI. The cavity created by HIFU is shown in the two-week post-treatment MRI (d).

contrast, showing encouraging accuracy in single centre studies (Figure 12.4).

Focal HIFU is currently being evaluated within phase II clinical studies with promising early results that demonstrate potency and continence rates of approximately 90-95% with 90% early cancer control. A larger prospective trial is necessary to assess the reproducibility and longer-term outcomes.

References

Ahmed HU, Zacharakis E, Dudderidge T, Armitage JN, Scott R, Calleary J, et al. High-intensity focused ultrasound in the treatment of primary prostate cancer: the first UK series. *Br J Cancer* 2009:**101**(1);19–26.

Madersbacher S, Pedevilla M, Vingers L, Susani M, Marberger M, Effect of high-intensity focused ultrasound on human prostate cancer in vivo. *Cancer Res* 1995;55:3346–51.

Murat F-J, Poissonnier L, Rabilloud M, Belot A, Bouvier R, Rouviere O, et al. Mid-term results demonstrate salvage high-intensity focused ultrasound (HIFU) as an effective and acceptably morbid salvage treatment option for locally recurrent prostate cancer. *Eur Urol* 2009:55:640–9.

Uchida T, Ohkusa H, Nagata Y, Hyodo T, Satoh T, Irie A. Treatment of localized prostate cancer using high-intensity focused ultrasound. *BJU Int* 2006:97:56–61.

Zacharakis E, Ahmed HU, Ishaq A, Scott R, Illing R, Freeman A, Allen C, Emberton M. The feasibility and safety of high-intensity focused ultrasound as salvage therapy for recurrent prostate cancer following external beam radiotherapy. *BJU Int* 2008;**102**(7);786–92.

Further reading

Ahmed HU, Pendse D, Illing R, Allen C, van der Meulen JH, Emberton M. Will focal therapy become a standard of care for men with localized prostate cancer? *Nat Clin Pract Oncol* 2007;**4**(11);632–42.

Illing RO, Leslie TA, Kennedy JE, Calleary JG, Ogden CW, Emberton M. Visually directed high-intensity focused ultrasound for organ-confined prostate cancer: A proposed standard for the conduct of therapy. *BJU Int* 2006:**98**:1187–92.

Kennedy JE, ter Haar GR, Cranston D. High intensity focused ultrasound: Surgery of the future? *Br J Radiol* 2003;**76**:590–9.

CHAPTER 13

Cryotherapy for Prostate Cancer

Alastair Henderson[1] *and John Davies*[2]

[1]Maidstone and Tunbridge Wells NHS Trust, Maidstone, Kent, UK
[2]University of Surrey, Guildford, UK

OVERVIEW

- Prostate cryotherapy may be used to treat primary organ confined or locally advanced prostate cancer and for salvage after failed radiotherapy

- The most established of the three roles is currently in radiation salvage treatment where cryotherapy is a leading minimally invasive treatment option

- The relative merits of primary treatment with cryotherapy for localised and locally advanced disease compared with other existing modalities has yet to be fully explored with comparative studies

- Contemporary randomised trials would be useful in each of the disease subgroups

- Focal cryotherapy is being explored as one of the 'male lumpectomy' options for controlling prostate cancer

---

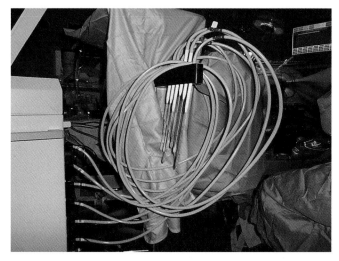

Figure 13.1 Iceball generated during cryoprobes testing prior to procedure.

Introduction

No single technology has become the definitive treatment for the most common of male malignancies. All of the current ablative technologies have advantages and problems. The terms cryosurgery and cryotherapy are used interchangeably in the literature and treatments may be described as whole gland or focal, depending on whether they aim to freeze the whole prostate or merely a section where foci of cancer have been detected. Primary treatment describes cryotherapy as a sole treatment whereas salvage treatments are usually applied where radiotherapy has already failed to control cancer.

The development of cryosurgery for prostate cancer

An awareness of the evolution of cryosurgical technology is critical when assessing the published literature as many historical treatment series used technology which generated much less controlled freezing with worse oncological and functional outcomes.

Current multi-probe argon-helium systems have evolved needles of increasingly small diameter (17-gauge). They utilise the Joule-Thompson effect which is a change in temperature, produced at the probe tip when high pressure gas is released to a lower pressure. The temperature at the probe tip may be reduced or increased depending on the physical properties of the gas chosen. Rapid cooling to temperatures as low as $-186°C$ may be achieved using Argon; Helium produces warming to temperatures of up to $40°C$. Figure 13.1 illustrates the iceball generated during probe testing on a modern device.

The availability of accurate thermocouples for continuous temperature monitoring of critical structures and the urethral warming catheter led to reductions in the significant complications of rectal fistulae and urethral sloughing which had been encountered in early cryotherapy. Constant improvement in the quality of trans-rectal ultrasound images due to the evolution of high definition multi-planar ultrasound arrays over the past 20 years has led to an ability to more accurately monitor the iceball and place the probes.

Mechanism of tissue injury in prostate cryotherapy

The aim of prostate cryotherapy is to destroy cancer and preserve vital structures around the prostate, including the bladder, rectum

---

and ideally the neurovascular bundles. This requires precise freezing. Two mechanisms are responsible for cell death: direct injury caused by ice formation and indirect ischemic effect caused by microvascular changes.

Physical measures of cold exposure have all been shown to affect cell viability post cryotherapy. These include rapidity of freezing, nadir temperatures of $-40°C$ in the double freeze cycle or $-61.7°C$ in the single freeze cycle, slow thawing rates, and increased length of exposure to freezing temperatures. A double freeze–thaw cycle achieving measured temperatures of $-40°C$ produces reliable cell kill which is not affected by tumour grade although higher grade tumours are more likely to be associated with occult micro-metastasis at presentation.

Patient groups amenable to total cryosurgical ablation of the prostate primary therapy – organ-confined disease

Organ-confined prostate cancer remains amenable to cryotherapy today although increasing competition from other treatment options means that this treatment is less frequently used for primary treatment compared with radiotherapy, brachytherapy and radical prostatectomy (see Chapters 10 and 11). Guidance was issued from the UK National Institute of Clinical Excellence (NICE 2005), based on their literature review which was prepared in 2004. This stated that in view of the current scarcity of evidence on the efficacy and safety of primary cryotherapy, it was not recommended for men with localised prostate cancer other than in the context of controlled clinical trials comparing their outcomes with those of more established interventions. The Cochrane Review Group (Shelley et al. 2007) considered cryotherapy for localised prostate cancer in 2007 and their findings supported these conclusions though further long-term case series have been published.

Primary therapy – locally advanced disease

Cryotherapy has been used to treat locally advanced prostate cancer where capsular penetration has occurred. A recent randomised controlled trial in T2c-T3b (bilateral organ confined, capsular penetration or seminal vesical invasion) by Chin et al. has suggested that biochemical disease-free survival was poorer in men who underwent cryotherapy as their primary treatment modality than in those who underwent primary External Beam Radiotherapy (EBRT). Clearly the subgroup of patients with capsular penetration and a contra-indication to EBRT may still wish to consider cryotherapy as primary therapy.

Salvage therapy after external beam radiotherapy or brachytherapy

The failure rates for contemporary EBRT in biochemical control of organ-confined prostate cancer range from 24–85% depending on the risk profile of the assessed group, the planning and delivery of radiotherapy and the length of follow-up. Due to the widespread use of EBRT often at lower radiation doses than are used currently, this group of patients is potentially the largest group of patients who are suitable for prostate cryotherapy. The workload of such patients who may require cryotherapy is also higher, in part due to the relative lack of other established modalities which are recognised as effective in the treatment of locally recurrent disease after radiotherapy. The other commonly used modality in this group in Europe is high intensity focused ultrasound (HIFU) (see Chapter 12) though no comparative randomised trials have been performed.

Patient selection for primary cryotherapy

As in patients undergoing primary treatment, a prostate volume of more than 40 cc^3 requires cytoreductive androgen deprivation in order to facilitate the procedure and reduce the risk to the surrounding structures. Use of established staging nomograms (as described by Roach or Partin) should be considered and the possibility of lymph node sampling considered if the chance of LN involvement is >15%.

Patient selection for salvage cryotherapy after EBRT or brachytherapy

If there is a persistent rise in PSA after radiotherapy which fulfils the Phoenix definition of biochemical failure (nadir PSA+ 2.0 mmol/dl), then staging investigations for salvage therapy may be instigated.

Urinary tract infection should be excluded. Restaging pelvic MRI scan and bone scan is necessary to exclude patients with metastatic disease prior to prostate biopsy. Prostate biopsy is mandatory to confirm local recurrence. Saturation prostate biopsy often using a brachytherapy template (20–40 cores) is more sensitive than trans-rectal biopsy (10 cores) in detection of recurrent cancer in irradiated patients. Cytoreductive androgen deprivation should be employed when prostate volume is >40cc and pelvic lymph node dissection is considered as in primary treatment.

Technique of cryosurgical ablation of the prostate

Figure 13.2 is a schematic of the modern cryotherapy technique. It illustrates the anaesthetised patient in the lithotomy position. The cryoprobes are placed via a perineal template. Temperature monitoring thermocouples are placed anterior to the rectum, in the anterior prostate, at the prostatic apex and in the urethral sphincter, all under ultrasound control. A urethral warmer is placed in a similar way to a catheter. Figure 13.3 shows an intraoperative photograph depicting the use of the template to secure the cryotherapy needles in place and a stepping unit to secure and manipulate the ultrasound probe.

Primary cryotherapy of the prostate

Biochemical recurrence-free survival (BRFS) rates of patients without a rising PSA after primary cryotherapy are variable, ranging from 60–90% at the last follow-up. Results depend on the era

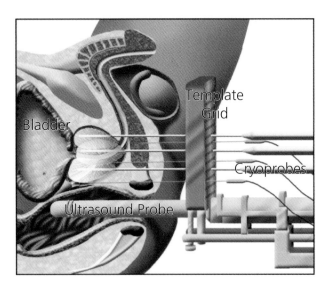

Figure 13.2 Schematic of prostate cryotherapy illustrates position of ultrasound probe in rectum to produce imaging guidance, cryoprobe and thermocouples held in situ by template with iceball covering prostate.

of the technology used, the severity of the cancer, the length of the follow-up and the criteria used in defining the cut-off for PSA recurrence. D'Amico risk groups stratify for disease severity; low-risk patients have no risk factors (from a PSA level ≤10 ng/ml,

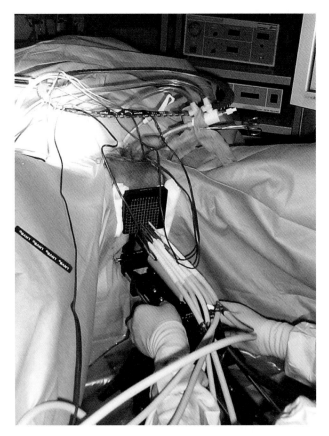

Figure 13.3 Set-up for prostate cryotherapy with urethral warmer in situ, black cryoprobes, and white thermocouples inserted via a perineal template.

a Gleason score ≤6 and a clinical stage ≤T2b) compared to intermediate with one risk factor and the high-risk patients with two or more unfavourable risk factors. In fact, 10-year actuarial BRFS rates of 81%, 74%, and 46% have been reported for the low-risk, intermediated-risk and high-risk groups respectively.

Complications of primary cryotherapy of the prostate

Complication rates are relatively low following primary prostate cryotherapy apart from erectile dysfunction which remains a common problem affecting 53–96% of men. Urinary incontinence rates varied considerably but were <10% in most series. Recto-urethral fistulae are an increasingly rare (<0.5% in reports from the last decade) though still potentially a very serious complication which may require diversion of urine or faeces using a stoma.

Oncological results of salvage cryotherapy series

Bahn et al. (2003) published a seven-year follow-up after salvage cryotherapy from 72 men with BRFS of 59–69%. Ten-year data published in 2010 on a mixed population of primary and salvage patients are available which showed a cancer-specific survival of 87%.

Complications of salvage cryotherapy series

Almost all patients following salvage cryotherapy will have some degree of lower urinary tract symptoms (LUTS) secondary to urethral slough, most of which will resolve in the first six months. In contemporary salvage cryotherapy series, the urinary incontinence rate has dropped dramatically with recent studies reporting incontinence rates of 3–6%.

The impotence rate in salvage cases ranges from 56–100%. In salvage cryotherapy, most patients suffer from a degree of pre-operative erectile dysfunction owing to previous hormone therapy and pelvic irradiation. Better controlled cryotherapy has significantly reduced recto-urethral fistula to <4% in salvage cases.

Focal nerve-sparing primary cryotherapy

In prostate cryotherapy, the whole prostate gland is frozen, including the peri-prostatic tissue with neurovascular bundles to eradicate all tumour cells. As a result, the incidence of erectile dysfunction is high. In an attempt to preserve potency, investigators have described focal nerve-sparing prostate cryotherapy where they treated part of the prostate which contains the tumour. Some 95% of the treated patients had stable PSA and 80% maintained their potency. In another series, 84% of patients had not experienced biochemical failure and only 14% showed positive biopsy on the treated site. Potency was maintained in 71% and no patient reported any worsening lower urinary tract symptoms or incontinence. Focal nerve-sparing cryotherapy has not been applied in salvage treatment.

References

Bahn DK, Lee F, Silverman P, Bahn E, Badalament R, Kumar A et al. Salvage cryosurgery for recurrent prostate cancer after radiation therapy: A seven-year follow-up. *Clin Prostate Cancer* 2003;**2**(2):111–14.

NICE. *Interventional Procedures Overview of Cryotherapy as a Primary Treatment for Prostate Cancer*. London: National Institute of Clinical Excellence, 2005:1–15.

Shelley M, Wilt TJ, Coles B, Mason MD. Cryotherapy for localised prostate cancer. *Cochrane Database Syst Rev* 2007(3):CD005010.

Further reading

Cohen JK, Miller RJ, Jr., Ahmed S, Lotz MJ, Baust J. Ten-year biochemical disease control for patients with prostate cancer treated with cryosurgery as primary therapy. *Urology* 2008;**71**(3):515–18.

Lambert EH, Bolte K, Masson P, Katz AE. Focal cryosurgery: encouraging health outcomes for unifocal prostate cancer. *Urology* 2007;**69**(6):1117–20.

CHAPTER 14

Advances in External Beam Radiotherapy

David Landau, Nadia Walsh and Asad Qureshi

Guy's and St Thomas' NHS Foundation Trust, London, UK

> ## OVERVIEW
>
> - The position of the prostate within the pelvis makes it susceptible to a range of movement over time with respect to surrounding fixed bony anatomy
> - Image guidance systems are used to enable visualisation of the treatment target within the body and provide the information to accurately align the patient to the correct position prior to treatment delivery
> - Intensity modulated radiotherapy is an advanced treatment delivery technique designed to sculpt the radiation dose closely to the shape of the treatment target while sparing surrounding normal tissues, thereby minimising treatment related side-effects
> - Image-guided techniques combined with intensity modulated RT facilitate safe escalation of the prescribed radiation dose to the target with minimal impact on toxicity, improving clinical outcomes

Introduction

The past decade has seen major advances in radiotherapy technology. Since higher-dose radiotherapy has been demonstrated to be of clinical benefit, prostate cancer is often the testing ground for new techniques. What defines a step forward in radiotherapy is an increased ability to avoid normal structures while still treating the whole of the target. The two methods for achieving this are improved localisation of the target and improved ability to shape the high radiation dose region more precisely to the shape of the target.

Advances in target localisation: image-guided radiotherapy (IGRT)

Cone beam CT (CBCT)

Having outlined the target (prostate +/- seminal vesicles and pelvic nodes) on CT images, the next step is to consider how to accurately locate the target daily. Prostate position varies in relation to the pelvic bony structures mainly as a result of variable rectal and bladder filling. The ability to perform a CT scan daily, immediately prior to treatment, allows the centre of the radiation beams (the isocentre) to be set to the correct position within the prostate each treatment.

Cone beam CT (CBCT) is a system that utilises diagnostic level 2D images via a kilovoltage X-ray source and image flat-panel mounted on the linear accelerator. This system rotates 360° around the patient, taking 500 to 600 images which are processed to produce a 3D image. This in turn is registered with the original planning CT in order to inform the radiographers how to shift the linear accelerator couch (and so the patient) to ensure that the isocentre is at the correct point in the target.

Studies using CBCT to assess prostate position prior to treatment have shown that a significant number of patients require a shift to improve accuracy of treatment (Wong et al. 2005). Using CBCT for online correction allows the margins used to account for organ motion to be reduced. Some studies have suggested it can be reduced from 10 mm to as little as 3 mm, which can lead to a reduced radiation dose to the rectum and reduced toxicity (Sandler et al. 2010).

As with all forms of IGRT discussed here, the impact on clinical outcome has not yet been finally determined, but the smaller treated volumes clearly result in less toxicity and allow for dose escalation and improved local control.

Fiducial markers

Another form of IGRT is the use of radio-opaque markers (often gold). At least three markers are placed in the prostate prior to the planning CT, usually a week earlier to allow the markers to settle in with no further subtle changes in position. The markers are imaged daily by either orthogonal megavoltage or kilovoltage beams. The combined images are processed and compared with the planning CT configuration to accurately reposition the treatment couch.

The process of marker insertion has been shown to be well tolerated with minimal complications. The most commonly seen side-effects are haematuria (0–15%), rectal bleeding (4–6.4%) and infection (3.2%) (Escudero et al. 2010). Using this system, systematic errors are reduced, allowing margins to be reduced by up to 4 mm. Studies comparing CBCT with implanted fiducial markers have shown equivalent set-up accuracy.

ABC of Prostate Cancer, First Edition.
Edited by Prokar Dasgupta and Roger S. Kirby.
© 2012 Blackwell Publishing Ltd. Published 2012 by Blackwell Publishing Ltd.

Radio-fiducials

Alternative systems are either available (e.g. Calypso) or in development that send real-time spatial information regarding prostate position using radiofrequency signals. As these are fiducial-based, they are very similar to those described above but differ in that no X-rays are required for positional information.

One immediate advantage of these systems over CBCT or radio-opaque fiducials is that they do not require repetitive CT imaging and hence save time and extra radiation dose to the patient. In addition, they can alert the radiographers to significant changes in position during treatment that might require the treatment to be stopped mid-fraction. A study of 20 patients showed that two patients had organ motion of >10 mm which could have led to geographic miss of the target. Comparison of radiofrequency tracking of implanted transponders with radiographic tracking shows minimal differences.

Advances in radiotherapy delivery

Intensity modulated radiotherapy (IMRT)

Conformal radiotherapy refers to the delivery of a number of radiation beams directed at the treatment target which are precisely shaped to the size and contour of the target volume in 3D. Beam shaping devices situated in the head of the linear accelerator, called multi-leaf collimators (MLC), are moved into the path of the beam to shield surrounding tissues (Figure 14.1a). IMRT is an advanced conformal radiotherapy technique which allows highly sculptured dose distributions around the target with rapid dose fall-off. The improved precision of IMRT treatment demands accuracy in target positioning as is now available with the IGRT

techniques described above. The clinician defines dose coverage parameters for the target and safe levels of irradiation to normal tissues. Using sophisticated software, these parameters are used to achieve an acceptable radiation dose distribution. In IMRT, the strength within each small area of the beam can change, as the MLCs move independently across the treatment beam to vary or 'modulate' the intensity. A fluence map (Figure 14.1b) describes the variation in intensity across the beam. This, usually together with an increase in the number and direction of radiation beams, allows much more control of the shape of the dose delivered. More specifically, concave-shaped dose distributions can be created to spare intimately associated critical structures, such as the rectum in relation to the prostate or the bladder and small bowel in relation to the pelvic nodes.

The clinical benefit of this technique is the potential to escalate the dose delivered and thereby improve local tumour control without impacting on late radiation toxicity. The UK MRC RT-01 trial randomly assigned men with localised prostate cancer to either 64Gy in 32 fractions or 74Gy in 37 fractions with conformal radiotherapy. The higher dose arm was associated with improved biochemical control and progression-free survival, however, it also showed an increase in rectal and bladder toxicity (Dearnaly et al. 2007). A US study delivered doses up to 81Gy with IMRT and IGRT while incidence of Grade 2 rectal toxicity remained low at 1.6% at eight years post treatment (Zelefsky et al. 2006).

There are two major disadvantages of IMRT technology. The first is the introduction of the 'low-dose bath' effect, whereby a low radiation dose is delivered to a larger cross-section of tissue, compared with standard conformal techniques. This may increase the likelihood of secondary cancers developing within the pelvis.

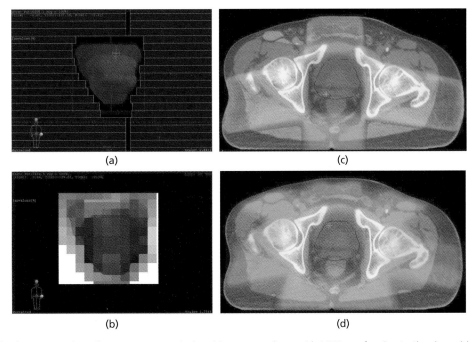

(a) (c)

(b) (d)

Figure 14.1 An anterior beam's eye-view of a prostate + seminal vesicles target volume with MLCs conforming to the shape (a), as used for conformal radiotherapy; (b) an IMRT fluence map showing varying intensities across the treatment beam; (c) 3D conformal dose distribution using a 3-field arrangement (d) IMRT dose distribution using a 7 beam arrangement which shows the red high-dose region to be better confined to the target area including a significantly reduced rectal dose.

The second is that due to the complex nature of IMRT, treatment delivery times are substantially increased, prolonging the time the patient spends on the treatment couch for each daily fraction. This impacts on the overall clinical capacity of radiotherapy departments.

Rotational IMRT

Rotational IMRT techniques improve the efficiency of treatment delivery. IMRT is delivered while the linear accelerator rotates around the patient, in one or more 360° arcs. The shape of the beam is continuously altered throughout the treatment to be optimal for each angle. Likewise the strength of the beam varies throughout the treatment. The result is a highly conformal distribution of radiation dose, at least equal to that achieved with fixed field IMRT. Arc therapy can currently be delivered in one of two ways: tomotherapy and volumetric arc therapy (VMAT).

Tomotherapy (literally 'slice therapy') uses a thin fan beam of radiation emitted from a source rotating 360° around the patient as they move through the machine and is best described as the combination of a linear accelerator and CT scanner. Helical tomotherapy (TomoTherapy® Inc., Madison, WI, USA) is a treatment system which combines IGRT and IMRT. CT detectors are mounted at 180° to the source, allowing the generation of CT images for IGRT. During treatment, detectors capture exit radiation to provide information about the dose actually delivered to the patient.

VMAT IMRT is delivered using a standard linear accelerator as it rotates around the patient. The entire treatment is generally delivered during one full gantry rotation, although in some more complex cases two arcs may be used to improve the dose distribution. The major advantage of VMAT is the increased efficiency of treatment delivery, compared with other forms of IMRT mentioned above. The 'low-dose bath' of radiation delivered to normal tissues is also reduced in comparison to fixed field IMRT.

CyberKnife®

CyberKnife® (Accuray, Sunnyvale, CA, USA) is an image-guided robotic stereotactic delivery system. A linear accelerator source is mounted onto a robotic arm, providing increased degrees of freedom for treatment delivery, further improving radiation dose conformity to the target. Stereotactic radiotherapy refers to the precise irradiation of a target using a small number of treatments with a large dose per fraction. Prostate cancers are thought to

have a greater sensitivity to radiation at higher doses per fraction (known as the α/β ratio) (Brenner et al. 2002). Stereotactic delivery allows large fraction sizes to be delivered with minimal toxicity to the rectum and bladder, which may lead to improvement in local control rates and overall survival compared with conventional dose fractionation regimens.

Particle therapy

Charged particles such as protons can be used in radiotherapy to provide an extremely focused radiation beam which deposits its energy at a predicted depth. Particles of a given energy have a certain range which results in no exit dose beyond the target. Due to their relatively large mass, protons also have little lateral scatter in tissue. Reduction of dose to normal tissues surrounding the target has the benefit of significantly minimising side-effects and reducing incidence of secondary cancers. The availability of particle therapy is extremely limited within the UK, and eligible patients must travel abroad to access treatment facilities.

References

Brenner DJ, Martinez AA, Edmundson GK, Mitchell C, Thames HD, Armour EP. Direct evidence that prostate tumors show high sensitivity to fractionation (low alpha/beta ratio), similar to late-responding normal tissue. *Int J Radiat Oncol Biol Phys.* 2002 Jan 1;**52**(1):6–13.

Dearnaly DP, Sydes MR, Graham JD, Aird EG, Bottomley D, Cowan RA et al. Escalated-dose versus standard-dose conformal radiotherapy in prostate cancer: first results from the MRC RT01 randomised controlled trial. *Lancet Oncology* 2007;**8**:475–87.

Escudero JU, Peidro JP, Campos MR, Torrecilla JL, Alcina EL, Verdejo PN et al. Insertion of intraprostatic gold fiducial markers in prostate cancer treatment. *International Journal of Nephrology and Urology* 2010;**2**: 265–72.

Sandler HM, Liu PY, Dunn RL, Khan DC, Tropper SE, Sanda MG et al. Reduction in patient-reported acute morbidity in prostate cancer patients treated with 81-Gy intensity-modulated radiotherapy using reduced planning target volume margins and electromagnetic tracking: Assessing the impact of margin reduction study. *J Urol* 2010;**75**:1004–8.

Wong J, Grimm L, Uematsu M, Oren R, Cheng CW, Merrick S et al. Image-guided radiotherapy for prostate cancer by CT-linear accelerator combination: prostate movements and dosimetric considerations. *IJROBP* 2005;**61**:561–9.

Zelefsky MJ, Chan H, Hunt M, Yamada Y, Shippy AM, Amols H. Long term outcome of high dose intensity modulated radiation therapy for patients with clinically localised prostate cancer. *J Urol* 2006;**176**:1415–19.

CHAPTER 15

Recent Advances in Hormonal Therapy

Heather Payne, Reena Davda and Mark R. Feneley

University College Hospital London, London, UK

OVERVIEW

- Hormonal therapy plays a key role in the treatment of prostate cancer
- Castration can be achieved with surgical orchidectomy or medical therapy with LHRHagonists or GnRH antagonists
- Castration-based therapy remains first line and mainstay treatment for men with advanced disease. It relieves symptoms and delays progression
- After a variable period of time, tumour growth can become resistant to testosterone depletion and other hormone manipulations can be added sequentially. These currently include anti-androgens, oestrogens and steroids
- New hormone therapies are under investigation and are showing great promise for castration-resistant prostate cancer. These include abiraterone acetate and MDV3100

Introduction

Hormonal therapy plays a key role in the treatment of prostate cancer. Huggins and Hodges first recognised the role of testosterone in stimulating prostate cancer cells in the early 1940s. Treatments aimed at lowering the serum testosterone then rapidly became established as effective management of advanced (metastatic) prostate cancer by reducing symptoms and slowing disease progression.

Since these early beginnings, there have been many advances in the hormone treatment of prostate cancer. Hormonal therapy now has an important role in the management of earlier stages of the disease, including its neoadjuvant and adjuvant combination with radical radiotherapy. New pharmacological approaches for targeting endocrine signalling pathways are in development.

Mode of action

In the early days, endocrine treatment of prostate cancer required the surgical removal of the testes, bilateral orchidectomy, thereby depleting circulating testosterone. Some 95% of serum testosterone is produced by the testes, without which low levels of androgens are maintained by the adrenal glands.

The first bilateral orchidectomy was performed in 1941 and still remains the gold standard against which all other hormonal therapies are judged. This surgical operation produces a rapid and sustained reduction in circulating testosterone within 12 hours. Although a very effective therapy, bilateral orchidectomy is non-reversible and can have an adverse psychological impact on many men.

The development of 'medical castration' using luteinising hormone-releasing hormone agonists (LHRHagonists) was a major breakthrough in the management of prostate cancer, introduced into clinical practice in the 1980s. Endogenous LHRH is produced by the neuroendocrine cells of the hypothalamus and causes the anterior pituitary to release luteinising hormone (LH) which in turn acts upon the Leydig cells of the testes, stimulating testosterone synthesis (Figure 15.1). Randomised studies have established that LHRHagonists are as effective as surgical castration, giving patients an important choice in the modality of their treatment.

The initial effect of treatment with LHRHagonist is a rise in serum testosterone. With ongoing or continuous treatment, the pituitary becomes depleted of LH and consequently testosterone falls to castrate levels by two weeks. This initial testosterone surge may theoretically result in a tumour flare. Until castrate levels are reached, the effect of testosterone can be dampened by preloading an anti-androgen (i.e. an androgen receptor blocker) prior to the first LHRHa injection, and continued for one to two weeks afterwards.

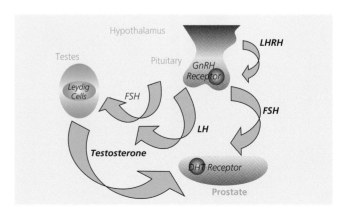

Figure 15.1 The hypothalamic-pituitary-gonadal axis.

ABC of Prostate Cancer, First Edition.
Edited by Prokar Dasgupta and Roger S. Kirby.
© 2012 Blackwell Publishing Ltd. Published 2012 by Blackwell Publishing Ltd.

A recent development in castration-based therapy has been the introduction of the gonadotrophin releasing hormone (GnRH) antagonists. These drugs bind competitively to GnRH receptors and produce a direct and rapid decline of LH, FSH and testosterone. When initiating treatment, there is no stimulation of GnRH, and therefore no testosterone surge and no clinical flare, so concurrent anti-androgen treatment is not required.

Anti-androgens such as bicalutamide and flutamide block the androgen receptor but not the production of testosterone. They have been shown to be equally effective as LHRH agonists injections for the treatment of locally advanced disease and have a different side effect profile.

Advanced prostate cancer

Hormonal manipulation with castration-based therapy remains first line and mainstay treatment for men with advanced (metastatic) disease. It relieves symptoms and delays progression. Response rates of over 85% can be expected for up to three years. The Medical Research Council (1997) study of immediate versus delayed hormonal therapy for metastatic prostate cancer (Figure 15.2) showed advantages for early treatment. Men treated with delayed hormones had significantly higher rates of spinal cord compression (Figure 15.3), pathological fracture, ureteric obstruction and extra-skeletal metastases. These findings support the introduction of early hormonal therapy prior to symptomatic progression.

After a variable period of time, tumour growth can become resistant to testosterone depletion. The addition of an anti-androgen to achieve combined androgen blockade (CAB) blocks the effect of residual testosterone on the androgen receptor with response rates of up to 30–50% for an average duration of six months. Subsequent withdrawal of the anti-androgen after relapse on CAB can result in further responses of 20–30%, with an overall duration of four to five months.

Other hormonal manipulations may be administered as sequential third and fourth line therapies. Diethylstilboestrol and or

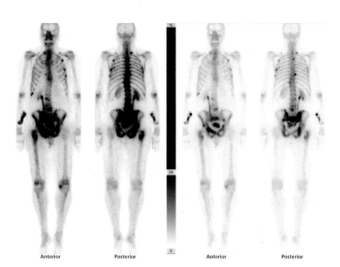

Figure 15.2 Bone scan showing bone metastases from prostate cancer. Source: Courtesy of Mr. John Anderson, Consultant Urologist, Royal Hallamshire Hospital, Sheffield.

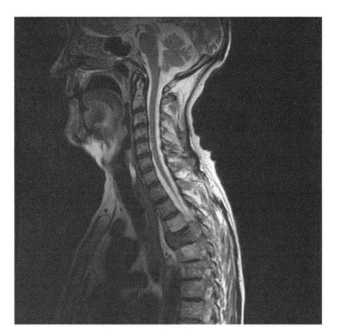

Figure 15.3 MRI scan showing spinal cord compression.

glucocorticoids can sometimes achieve further remission for up to six months or longer. Oestrogen therapy is associated with gynaecomastia, fluid retention and thrombo-embolism. Cardiovascular events can be prevented with aspirin or anticoagulants. By these means, various endocrine signalling pathways can be targeted to delay progression of advanced prostate cancer, indicating hormone-dependent activity in spite of low levels of circulating androgen.

There are many new hormone compounds under investigation which are showing great promise for the future. Tumour resistance to testosterone depletion develops in the course of malignant progression through phenotypic selection of the most aggressive cells. In spite of their so-called hormone resistance to androgen deprivation therapy, prostate cancer often continues to be androgen-driven. High concentration of androgens can be demonstrated in tumour tissue in spite of castrate levels of serum testosterone, indicating androgen synthesis within the tumour.

Abiraterone acetate is a potent, selective inhibitor of CYP17, key enzymes in androgen synthesis, and completely blocks the production of testosterone. Clinical trials have shown encouraging results in men with castrate-resistant prostate cancer (CRPC), with up to 67% demonstrating a PSA response.

It is also known that the androgen receptor may be activated despite very low levels of testosterone. Prostate cancer progression is associated with androgen receptor amplification or over-expression, and mutation; either or both of these mechanisms may increase tumour sensitivity to androgens and anti-androgens. The functional activity of the testosterone-bound androgen receptor is also regulated by binding of co-activators and co-pressors. In advanced malignancy, androgen receptor activity may be enhanced through altered availability of these co-factors and abnormal intracellular signalling. Mechanisms also exist for androgen independent androgen receptor activation.

MDV3100 is a new oral androgen receptor antagonist that inhibits its nuclear translocation and blocks its binding with DNA.

This drug has shown great promise in trials of men with CRPC, and PSA responses of 55% have been seen in chemotherapy naïve patients and 36% in those previously treated with docetaxel. These two new compounds, Abiraterone and MDV3100, are currently being investigated in large randomised Phase III studies and the results of these trials are awaited with great interest.

Neoadjuvant and adjuvant hormonal therapy

Hormonal therapy has evolved to play a critical role in the management of prostate cancer that is locally advanced or clinically localised but so-called 'high risk' (Gleason Grade ≥8, PSA ≥20), as combination treatment with radical radiotherapy. In these patients the therapeutic challenges reflect the need to control local disease as well as subclinical microscopic distant metastases. Traditional treatment with external beam radiotherapy alone frequently fails to prevent distant progression, despite improvements in radiotherapy dose and delivery, owing to undetectable micro-metastatic disease at diagnosis. There is a wealth of data to support the addition of systemic hormonal therapy which is now considered standard of care for men with high risk prostate cancer.

Neoadjuvant hormonal therapy, (with a LHRHagonist) is commonly used for two to three months prior to definitive radiotherapy This reduces the size of the prostate by an average of 25–30% which potentially allows smaller fields of radiotherapy to be used with some sparing of the rectum and bladder volumes and potentially reduced toxicity. There are reports that there may also be a sensitising effect between hormonal therapy and radiation treatment. This combination has been shown to demonstrate a significant improvement in disease-free survival in clinical studies.

There is strong supporting evidence for continued adjuvant hormone treatment after radical radiotherapy. A study by Bolla et al. (2008) reported that, in patients with locally advanced prostate cancer, LHRHagonist (goserelin) therapy initiated with radiotherapy and continued for three years improved overall survival compared with hormonal therapy deferred until disease progression. A recent update of this trial reported an 18.3% improvement in 10-year overall survival (58.1% vs 39.8% respectively). There were similar significant improvements for progression free survival and clinical or PSA relapse. Other randomised Phase III studies of adjuvant LHRHagonists have demonstrated similar benefit, and adjuvant antiandrogen therapy with bicalutamide 150 mg has also been shown to improve survival. It is now standard practice for hormone treatment to be continued for two to three years after radiotherapy.

Side-effects of hormonal therapy

The main toxicities of hormone treatment with LHRHagonists are shown in Table 15.1. These side-effects need to be balanced with the benefits of therapy as described above. The potential risks of treatment should be discussed with all men embarking on hormonal therapy for early detection of toxicities and intervention. The anti-androgens (e.g. bicalutamide 150 mg) have some advantages over castration-based therapy in that they can maintain physical capacity and bone mineral density (through aromatisation

Table 15.1 Side-effects of hormonal therapy.

Erectile dysfunction
Reduced libido
Osteopaenia/osteoporosis
Reduced muscle mass
Breast swelling and mastalgia
Weight gain
Hot flushes
Lethargy
Anaemia
Mood swings and depression
Metabolic complications, e.g. insulin resistance, hypertension and alterations in lipid levels

of available testosterone to oestrogen in bone) with lesser risk of hot flushes and loss of sexual function. However, they carry a greater risk of gynaecomastia and mastalgia. The different side-effect profiles of these two types of hormonal therapy can allow clinicians and patients to choose the best approach to maintain quality of life while assuring effective oncological therapy for the individual.

Conclusion

Hormonal therapy has remained a gold standard in the management of prostate cancer for more than 60 years. This has evolved from surgical to medical castration with the introduction of the LHRH agonists and more recently GnRH antagonists. Through advances in the use of hormonal therapy, treatment intent has evolved from purely palliative in advanced (metastatic) prostate cancer to now potentially curative by combination with radiotherapy in locally advanced disease. The therapeutic possibilities are likely to increase in the near future as we await the results of clinical trials of new and promising hormone therapies.

References

Bolla M, Collette L, Van Tienhoven G et al. Ten year results of long term adjuvant androgen deprivation with goserelin in patients with locally advanced prostate cancer treated with radiotherapy: A phase III EORTC study. *Int J Radiat Oncol Biol Phys* 2008;**72**(1 Suppl1): S30-S31.

The Medical Research Council Prostate Cancer Working Party Investigators Group Immediate versus deferred treatment for advanced prostatic cancer: initial results of the Medical Research Council Trial. *Br J Urol* 1997;**79**:235–46.

Further reading

Attard G et al. Selective inhibition of CYP17 with arbiraterone acetate is highly active in castrate resistant prostate cancer. *J Clin Oncol* 2009;**27**(23):3742–8. Epub 2009 May 26.

McLeod DG, Iversen P, See WA, Morris T, Armstrong J, Wirth M, on behalf of the Casodex Early Prostate Cancer Trialists' Group. Bicalutamide 150mg plus standard care vs standard care alone for early prostate cancer. *BJU International* 2005;**97**:247–54.

Pilepich MV, Winter K, Lawton CA, Krisch RE, Wolkov HB, Movsas B et al. A ndrogen suppression adjuvant to definitive radiotherapy in prostate carcinoma – long-term results of phase III RTOG 85-31. *Int J Radiat Oncol Biol Phys* 2005;**61**(5):1285–90.

CHAPTER 16

Management of Castration-Resistant Prostate Cancer

Roger S. Kirby[1], *Prokar Dasgupta*[2] *and John M. Fitzpatrick*[3]

[1] The Prostate Centre, London, UK
[2] Department of Urology, King's College London, Guy's and St Thomas' Hospital NHS Foundation Trust, London, UK
[3] UCD School of Medicine and Medical Science, Mater Misericordiae University Hospital, University College Dublin, Dublin, Ireland

OVERVIEW

- There is new hope for patients with castrate-resistant prostate cancer
- Docetaxel-based chemotherapy can improve survival in some patients
- Cabazitaxel is a new generation taxane for docetaxel-resistant patients
- Abiraterone has shown promising results in Phase II and III trials
- Sipuleucel-T is the first active immunotherapy to demonstrate an improvement in overall survival for advanced prostate cancer

Introduction

The survival of men with castration-resistant prostate cancer (CRPC) has generally been regarded as poor. However, the median survival in recent Phase III studies has ranged from 12.2 to 21.7 months, with improvements in survival seen mostly with docetaxel-based regimens. Two publications, both appearing in 2004, firmly established the benefits of this therapy. In the landmark TAX-327 trial, 1006 chemotherapy-naïve CRPC patients were randomised to three different treatment arms: docetaxel 30 mg/m^2 every week, docetaxel 75 mg/m^2 every three weeks and mitoxantrone 12 mg/m^2 every three weeks. All patients received prednisone 5 mg orally twice a day. Patients receiving docetaxel every three weeks had a significant improvement of survival compared to weekly docetaxel and mitoxantrone (18.9 months vs 16.5 months; $p < 0.009$). PSA response, pain control and quality of life were also significantly better with docetaxel every three weeks compared to mitoxantrone. An update of the results of TAX-327 trial published in 2007 showed a survival benefit of docetaxel every three weeks compared to mitoxantrone and no survival benefit with the weekly docetaxel. At three years, survival was 17.2% for docetaxel every three weeks compared to 12.8% with mitoxantrone ($p = 0.005$).

The Southwest Oncology Group (SWOG) 99-16 study also shows survival benefit with docetaxel. Some 674 patients with metastatic CRPC were randomised to docetaxel/estramustine and mitoxantrone/prednisone arms. Treatment regimen was 280 mg of estramustine three times daily on days 1 through 5, docetaxel 60 mg/m^2 on day 2 in the docetaxel arm and 12 mg of mitoxantrone mg/m^2 on day 1 plus 5 mg of prednisone twice daily in the mitoxantrone arm. Docetaxel was reported to be superior to mitoxantrone with a median survival of 17.5 months vs 15.6 months ($p = 0.02$), median time to progression (6.3 vs 3.2 months; $p < 0.001$) and PSA declines of 50% (50% vs 27%; $p < 0.001$). These two trials showed a 20–24% reduction in mortality in patients with CRPC treated with docetaxel-based chemotherapy.

There is now new hope for patients who relapse following docetaxel-based therapy. Until recently, treatment was only palliative, as no therapy had been shown to produce a survival benefit in this setting. However, a new generation taxane, cabazitaxel, has been developed to overcome docetaxel resistance, and is now available in the USA, and hopefully soon in Europe. Cabazitaxel, similar to docetaxel, is a semi-synthetic microtubule stabiliser extracted from needles of the European yew tree. In pre-clinical studies, cabazitaxel offers the advantage of being active *in vitro* and *in vivo* in cell lines and tumour models resistant to docetaxel, and shows a better blood–brain barrier penetration than other taxanes. In tumour models sensitive to docetaxel, its anti-tumour activity is comparable to docetaxel. In a large Phase III trial, 755 patients with metastatic CRPC progressing during or after docetaxel treatment were randomised to receive cabazitaxel (25 mg/m^2 every three weeks) plus prednisone/prednisolone (10 mg daily) or mitoxantrone (12 mg/m^2 every three weeks) plus prednisone/prednisolone, an active treatment commonly used for palliation at this stage of the disease. Primary end-point was overall survival. Cabazitaxel significantly reduced the risk of death by 30% (HR = 0.70, 95%CI [0.59–0.83]; $p < 0.0001$) with a median overall survival of 15.1 months versus 12.7 months with mitoxantrone. Progression-free survival, tumour response and PSA response were also significantly improved with cabazitaxel compared to mitoxantrone. In this population with very advanced disease and heavily pre-treated with chemotherapy, the most frequent grade 3/4 adverse events observed with cabazitaxel compared to mitoxantrone were neutropenia (81.7% vs 58%), febrile neutropenia (7.5% vs 1.3%) and diarrhoea (6.2% vs 0.3%). Patients should be carefully monitored for these adverse events, especially at treatment initiation, but if they occur they are readily manageable.

ABC of Prostate Cancer, First Edition.
Edited by Prokar Dasgupta and Roger S. Kirby.
© 2012 Blackwell Publishing Ltd. Published 2012 by Blackwell Publishing Ltd.

The prospects for further improvements in survival for men with CRPC are even more promising, considering that several molecules targeting angiogenesis (aflibercept), endothelin receptor (atrasentan, zibotentan), steroid receptor coactivator (dasatinib), RANK Ligand (denosumab) and immune response (sipuleucel-T, prost-vac VF) are either in late stage of development (Phase III) or actually launched (sipuleucel-T). These have been the subject of a recent review, however, shortage of space precludes the possibility of discussing all of them here. Sipuleucel as immunotherapy is particularly expensive ($98,000) and is discussed elsewhere in this book (Chapter 18).

Among a number of novel targets being evaluated are several endothelin-receptor antagonists. Endothelins (endothelin-1, endothelin-2, and endothelin-3) are regulators of cell proliferation, vasomotor tone, and angiogenesis. The endothelins bind to two receptors, endothelin-A and endothelin-B, and play a major role in tumour growth, proliferation, apoptosis, angiogenesis, and bone metastasis. Patients with metastatic prostate cancer have elevated levels of plasma endothelin-1 compared with patients with organ-confined cancer. Endothelin-A is thought to promote osteoblastic activity characteristic of bone metastases in prostate cancer.

Atrasentan, predominantly an endothelin-A receptor antagonist, was studied in two Phase III trials. In the first study, 809 patients with CRPC were randomised to atrasentan 10 mg daily vs placebo. The primary endpoints were time-to-progression (TTP) which was determined according to radiographic and clinical measures. Atrasentan did not reduce the risk of disease progression relative to the placebo (hazard ratio, 0.89; $p = 0.136$). In exploratory analyses, however, bone alkaline phosphatase and PSA levels were significantly lower in the atrasentan arm. Atrasentan generally was tolerated well, and the most common adverse events associated with treatment were headache, rhinitis, and peripheral edema, reflecting the vasodilatory and fluid-retention properties of endothelin-A receptor blockade. In a second Phase III trial, 941 men with PSA-only CRPC were randomised to receive atrasentan 10 mg daily vs placebo.

Although not statistically significant, fewer patients treated with atrasentan experienced disease progression compared with placebo ($p = 0.288$) and the median survival was longer for the atrasentan group ($p = 0.176$). Although it did not meet the primary endpoint expectations, atrasentan did have an impact on molecular markers that indicate disease progression. There was improvement in bone alkaline phosphatase (-1.51 IU/L (A) vs +2.2 IU/l (P); $p = 0.001$) and PSA doubling time was delayed ($p = 0.031$). An ongoing Phase III study, the Southwest Oncology Group trial (SWOG S0421) is evaluating atrasentan in combination with docetaxel/prednisone as a first-line treatment in metastatic CRPC.

Zibotentan (ZD4054) is a specific endothelin A (ET_A) receptor antagonist that unlike atrasentan has no detectable activity at the endothelin B (ET_B) receptor. The results of early clinical trials supported a large Phase II trial in men with CRPC. A randomised, double-blind, placebo-controlled, parallel-group, Phase II trial was undertaken in 65 centres in 14 countries across Europe, North America, Australasia and South East Asia. A total of 312 patients with HRPC and bone metastases who were pain free or mildly symptomatic for pain were recruited and randomised to receive once daily zibotentan 10 mg (n = 107), or 15 mg (n = 98), or matching placebo (n = 107). The primary endpoint was time to progression, defined as clinical progression, requirement for opiate analgesia, objective progression of soft-tissue metastases, or death in the absence of progression. PSA progression and change in number or appearance of bone metastases on scintigraphic imaging did not count as progression events. Secondary endpoints included overall survival, PSA progression, and safety.

At the primary analysis, no statistically significant difference in time to progression was observed for zibotentan versus placebo (HR: 10 mg, 0.88 [80% CI 0.71, 1.09]; 15 mg, 0.83 [0.66, 1.03]). However, a promising signal for prolonged overall survival was observed in the zibotentan treatment groups versus placebo, based on 40 deaths (HR: zibotentan 10 mg, 0.38 [80% CI 0.22, 0.64], $p = 0.019$; zibotentan 15 mg, 0.61 [0.38, 0.99], $p = 0.190$). At the second analysis, after 118 deaths, the survival benefit was sustained (HR versus placebo: zibotentan 10 mg, 0.55 [80% CI 0.41, 0.73], $p = 0.008$; zibotentan 15 mg, 0.65 [0.49, 0.86], $p = 0.052$), while there continued to be no significant difference in time to progression. Median overall survival was 24.5 and 23.5 months in the zibotentan 10 mg and 15 mg treatment groups, respectively, compared with 17.3 months in the placebo group. At the final analysis, a total of 211 (68%) deaths had occurred. There was a promising signal for overall survival (HR versus placebo: zibotentan 10 mg, 0.83 [80% CI 0.67, 1.02], $p = 0.254$; zibotentan 15 mg, 0.76 [0.61, 0.94], $p = 0.103$), while there continued to be no significant difference in time to progression. Median overall survival was 24.5 and 23.5 months in the zibotentan 10 mg and 15 mg treatment groups, respectively, compared with 17.3 months in the placebo group. Consistent with the previous analyses, no statistically significant differences were observed in TTP for either zibotentan 15 mg compared with placebo (HR 0.86, 80% CI: 0.72–1.04, $p = 0.309$) or zibotentan 10 mg compared with placebo (HR 1.06, 80% CI: 0.89–1.27, $p = 0.673$) at the final analysis. No significant differences were observed in time to PSA progression. Adverse events were in line with the expected pharmacodynamic effects of an ET_A receptor antagonist, most commonly headache, peripheral oedema and nasal congestion.

The promising improvement in overall survival with zibotentan seen in the Phase II study supports further investigation in Phase III clinical trials, with overall survival as the primary endpoint. The zibotentan ENdoTHelin A inhibitor USE (ENTHUSE) Phase III clinical trial programme consists of three randomised, double-blind trials, which together will include more than 3000 patients with HRPC across more than 400 centres worldwide.

There is also considerable anticipation, and a good deal of media coverage, concerning the prospects for abiraterone. Several preclinical and clinical studies have shown that despite being 'hormone refractory', prostate cancer cells continue to express high androgen receptor expression and thus mediate androgen signalling. Abiraterone acetate is a potent and a highly selective irreversible inhibitor of cytochrome P-17 (17 a hydroxylase and C17,20-lyase), a dual enzyme that blocks adrenal androgen production.

In a study, 58 patients who had progressive, metastatic CRPC and had failed hormonal therapy and up to two cytotoxic regimens, including docetaxel, were treated with abiraterone (1,000 mg once daily) and prednisone (5 mg twice daily). Twenty-five of 56 patients (45%) had a PSA decline ≥50%. Median time to PSA progression was 169 days. The majority of abiraterone-related adverse events were grades 1–2 and no grade 4 adverse events were reported. Also noted was a significantly better PSA response in the ketoconazole-naïve post-docetaxel CRPC population. A randomised Phase III pivotal study to confirm these results is ongoing.

Recent evidence has also indicated an important role for vaccine-based immunotherapy in CRPC. Sipuleucel-T (Provenge) consists of autologous peripheral blood mononuclear cells, including antigen presenting cells, that have been activated during a defined culture period with a recombinant fusion protein consisting of prostatic acid phosphatase (PAP), an antigen expressed in prostate cancer tissue, linked to granulocyte-macrophage colony-stimulating factor (GM-CSF), an immune cell activator. The patient's peripheral blood mononuclear cells are obtained via a standard leukapheresis procedure approximately three days prior to the infusion date. The active components are autologous antigen presenting cells and human PAP-GM-CSF fusion protein. During culture, the recombinant antigen can bind to and be processed by antigen presenting cells into smaller protein fragments. The recombinant antigen is designed to target antigen presenting cells, and may help direct the immune response to PAP. Minimal residual levels of the intact human PAP-GM-CSF fusion protein are detectable in the final sipuleucel-T product. The cellular composition of sipuleucel-T is dependent on the composition of cells obtained from the patient's leukapheresis. The activated, antigen-loaded APCs are then infused into the patient, where it can potentially stimulate a T cell response against prostate cancer cells. The process is performed three times over the course of a four-week period. The vaccine has been studied in three Phase III clinical trials. In the first Phase III study, D9901, consisting of 127 men with asymptomatic, metastatic CRPC, sipuleucel-T every two weeks for three cycles was compared with placebo in a 2:1 ratio. The final three-year follow-up of the D9901 phase III study showed a median survival benefit of 4.5 months and a threefold improvement in survival at 36 months for patients who were randomised to receive Provenge. In another similar phase III trial, D9902A, 98 men with asymptomatic, metastatic CRPC demonstrated a 21.4% improvement in overall survival (OS) for patients randomised to sipuleucel-T. In both studies, the vaccine was well tolerated, and the most common adverse events were chills and fatigue. The third Phase III trial, D9902B, also known as the IMPACT trial (Immunotherapy for Prostate Adenocarcinoma Treatment) was a randomised, double-blind, placebo-controlled study comparing Provenge with placebo in 512 men with CRPC randomised in 2:1 ratio. The median overall survival favoured the vaccine arm with a 4.1-month increase in overall survival for patients treated with sipuleucel-T (25.8 vs 21.7 months; $p = 0.032$). Also, the 36-month survival probability was 31.7% in the sipuleucel-T group versus 23.0% in the placebo group. Therapy with sipuleucel-T was also associated with a positive overall survival effect in an analysis that included 18 additional deaths observed between the data-cutoff and study-completion dates, with a median of 36.5 months of follow-up (hazard ratio, 0.76; 95% CI, 0.61 to 0.95; $p = 0.02$). Sipuleucel-T is the first active immunotherapy to demonstrate an improvement in overall survival for advanced prostate cancer. Given the short duration of the therapy (one month) and its favourable benefit-to-risk ratio, sipuleucel-T provides an attractive new option for the management of advanced prostate cancer.

Conclusion

In conclusion, a number of promising avenues are now available for men with CRPC. For the present, chemotherapy with docetaxel provides the mainstay, but newer options, including abiratarone, seem promising and are likely to be added to the armamentarium shortly.

Further reading

De Bono JS, Oudard S., Ozguroglu M. et al. Cabazitaxel or mitoxantrone with prednisone in patients with metastatic castration-resistant prostate cancer (mCRPC) previously treated with docetaxel: Final results of a multinational phase III trial (TROPIC). *J. Clin Oncol* 2010;**28**(suppl): 4508.

James, N.D., Caty, A., Borre, M. et al. Safety and efficacy of the specific endothelin A receptor antagonist ZD4054 in patients with hormone-resistant prostate cancer and bone metastases who were pain free or mildly symptomatic: A double-blind, placebo-controlled, randomized, Phase II trial. *Eur Urol* 2009;**55**:1112–23.

Kantoff P, Higano C, Shore D, et al. Sipuleucel-t immunotherapy for castration-resistant prostate cancer. *N Engl J Med* 2010;**363**:411–21.

Kirby RS, Fitzpatrick J. Improved survival prospects for men with castration resistant prostate cancer. *BJUInt* 2011 (in press).

Saad F, Gleason DM, Murray R, et al. A randomised, placebo-controlled trial of zoledronic acid in patients with hormone refractory metastatic prostate carcinoma. *J Natl Cancer Inst* 2002;**94**:1458–68.

Acknowledgements

The authors acknowledge the BJU International. PDG acknowledges support from the MRC Centre for Transplantation, NIHR Biomedical Research Centre.

CHAPTER 17

Immunology of Prostate Cancer

Oussama Elhage[1], *Christine Galustian*[1], *Richard Smith*[1] and *Prokar Dasgupta*[2]

[1]King's College London, London, UK
[2]Department of Urology, King's College London, Guy's and St Thomas' Hospital NHS Foundation Trust, London, UK

OVERVIEW

- Immunoediting is a process in which tumours are eliminated by the immune system in the initial phase, then followed by the equilibrium phase and finally by the escape phase when tumours evade immune control. This is the currently held hypothesis on the interaction between cancer and the immune system

- The prostate gland is a poorly immunogenic gland, however, it has a set of distinct antigens (PSA, PSMA, PAP) that can be exploited to be used for immunotherapy treatment

- Cancer immunotherapy strategy aims at stimulating the adaptive immune system to attack cancer cells. An organ-specific tumour antigen or group of antigens can be used to 'show' and 'teach' the immune system where and what to attack

- There are various ways to present these antigens to the immune system. The only FDA-approved treatment is sipuleucel which uses the patient's own dentritic cells (DC) to load PAP antigen onto the antigen-loaded DC cells in the patient. This then elicit an anti-tumour immune response extending the life of patients by 4.5 months on average

- All immunotherapy approaches so far have concentrated on treating patients with metastatic prostate cancer whose immune system is 'fatigued'. A treatment strategy aiming at treating early cancer would exploit a better functioning immune system

Prostate cancer and the immune system

The concept that the immune system can combat cancer was put forward over 100 years ago with the discovery that immune effector cells can recognise cancer cells as non-self, and thus can eliminate them in the same way as viral or microbial pathogens. Both the innate immune system consisting of non-antigen-specific cells such as macrophages, dendritic cells, neutrophils, natural killer cells, gamma delta T cells, and complement, and the adaptive immune system, with antigen-specific cytotoxic and helper T cells and antibody-producing B cells which can obtain a memory phenotype against specific antigenic challenge, are known to be able to respond

Table 17.1 Type of tumour-associated antigens.

Type of tumour-associated antigens	Example in prostate
Unique point mutation-specific tumour antigens	Spas-1
Tumour-specific antigens	Cancer–testis antigens e.g. NY-ESO1
Over-expressed antigens (greater expression in tumour vs normal tissue)	GAD1, CARM-1, PSMA, PSA, Dickkopf-1
Viral antigens	XMRV

against cancer cells, through the ability to recognise them as foreign. For example, many tumour antigens are known to be recognised by T cells and B cells and both tumour antigen-specific T cells and antibodies against tumour antigens can be detected in patients with cancers such as melanoma, ovarian cancer, colorectal carcinoma, and hepatocellular cell carcinoma. These antigens fall into a number of types including unique patient or shared tumour-specific antigens, antigens which are in both tumours and normal tissues, and viral antigens. In prostate cancer, a number of antigens are also known to be expressed which can be used for prostate cancer diagnosis or monitoring (Table 17.1).

The stages of tumour elimination by the immune system follow a pattern where there is an initial recruitment of immune cells including either neutrophils, monocytes and macrophages to the site of the tumour, normally through the presence of acute or chronic pro-inflammatory signals which are produced by normal or tumour cells reacting to the tumour micro-environment. These cells release cytokines and chemokines such as IL-8 and IL-6 which will attract T cells and NK cells to the sites of the tumour. Inflamed endothelium in these areas also express E-selectin, which will recruit cells such as T and B lymphocytes and neutrophils which express carbohydrate ligands such as Lewis x and sialyl Lewis X. Once T cells and NK cells can get to the tumour, they will secrete other chemokines and cytokines such as interferon gamma and IL-2 and IL-12 for further recruitment of T cells, NK cells, B cells and Dendritic cells, and these are critical in taking up antigens for presentation to helper T cells in the lymph nodes for the creation of antigen-specific T cells, and for the creation of an antibody response against the tumour antigens. B cells also take up antigen

ABC of Prostate Cancer, First Edition.
Edited by Prokar Dasgupta and Roger S. Kirby.
© 2012 Blackwell Publishing Ltd. Published 2012 by Blackwell Publishing Ltd.

for processing either through T cells or independently, and can process antigen for antibody production. During the last stages of the elimination phase the tumour-specific CD4 helper and CD8 cytotoxic T lymphocytes from the lymph nodes and tumour specific antibodies infiltrate the tumour environment to eliminate the tumour cells, with some antibodies acting through ADCC (antibody dependent cellular cytotoxicity) via Fc receptors on NK cells.

The concept of immunoediting

In prostate cancer, as in many other cancers, the concept of tumour elimination by the immune system has been superseded by a new hypothesis, known as immunoediting. In this hypothesis, there is the initial phase described above where the immune system can recognise and actively react and eliminate tumour cells appearing within a normal tissue environment, however, there are two further phases known as equilibrium, and escape.

In the equilibrium phase, there is a balance between the destruction of tumour cells by the immune system and the proliferation of new tumour cells in the lesion. The new cells formed are eliminated in due course, but the immune system cannot eliminate the lesion completely. In prostate cancer and breast cancer, this phase may last for many years with either a minimal residual tumour volume obtained after surgery or radiotherapy or with small tumours that are non palpable and therefore not detectable for many years. The reasons for this equilibrium state are as yet unclear, however, the coexistence of tumour cells with immune cells has been observed in a number of animal models.

The third stage of the hypothesis is escape. In this phase, cells may be growing at a rapid or slow rate, but these cells are now able to evade the immune system by one or more of a number of techniques such as the production of factors to prevent attack or masking of the cell surface by a loss or alteration of surface antigens such as MHC molecules, or the ability to move away from the site of capture (metastasis). Such cells that are growing in the presence of an ongoing immune response have either grown to resist the immune onslaught by selective pressure or have an inherent or induced genetic predisposition to evade recognition, or to inhibit the effector cells that they encounter.

Factors that cause immunosuppression in prostate cancer

There is an immense arsenal of immunosuppressive factors that the tumour cells themselves or the cells or stroma of the tumour microenvironment are able to produce to enable the continued existence of a cancer population. The micro-environment of the cancerous prostate has been shown to be very immunosuppressive and prostate cancer cells are frequently poorly immunogenic, i.e. unable to give rise to an immune response.

Suppressive immune cell populations within the prostate tumour environment

Although the infiltration of functionally active lymphocytes into tumour lesions is a favourable state for the elimination of the tumour cells, in high grade prostate cancer, immune infiltrates of CD3+ T cells are significantly diminished. Also immune infiltrates have been shown to frequently consist of anergic or suppressive T cell populations such as CD4+CD25+FOXP3+ regulatory T cells (known as Tregs) and also a rarer CD8+CD25+FOXP3 + population. Both these cell types suppress both T cell proliferation and activity and NK function. Other suppressor populations appearing in the infiltrate are myeloid suppressor cells. These are immature myeloid cells which are either resident in the tissue or migrate there through recruitment, but have a suppressor function against dendritic cells, T cells and NK cells in the tissue. The phenotype of these cells is not well characterised, but is thought to consist of Cd33+CD11b positive cells. The suppressive cells are either recruited into the tumour lesion by chemokines secreted by the tumour itself, or they are formed from active non-suppressive effector cell populations through the functions of cytokines secreted from the tumour or stromal tissue. For example, prostate cancer cells and the cells of their surrounding environment such as fibroblasts, can secrete TGF beta, IL-2 and IL-10 which can actively induce the production of Tregs and myeloid suppressor cells. Although Tregs can naturally occur in the immune system, they are of thymic origin and therefore as the thymus is absent or atrophied in old age, the Tregs of prostate cancer patients (who are diagnosed later in life) are thought to be induced in the tumour environment itself. The molecule indoleamine 2,3-dioxygenase (IDO) secreted by myeloid suppressor cells and by fibroblasts and other stromal components also suppresses T cell and NK cell function.

Suppressive stromal proteins in the prostate tumour environment

A number of suppressive prostate associated proteins have also been discovered, for example, fibroblast associated protein (FAP-1). These proteins are secreted in the normal prostate microenvironment but higher levels are associated with cancerous stroma. Their inhibitory functions have not been well characterised, but they can inhibit proliferation and the function of effector T cells and NK cells.

Loss of antigenic and gain of inhibitory tumour membrane bound proteins

A complement attack of tumour cells can happen through direct antibody involvement or through ADCC mechanisms, as described previously. The inhibition of complement by tumour cells is an evasive mechanism which attenuates the effects of antibodies toward tumour antigens and also may reduce the efficacy of antibody therapies such as herceptin. Membrane-bound complement regulatory proteins such as CD46, CD59, CD55 and CD97 (a receptor for CD55) are known to be expressed frequently in tumour cell populations and the receptors CD55 and CD97 are upregulated in prostate cancer biopsies from primary and metastatic disease and in patients with prostate interstitial neoplasia (PIN) compared to biopsies from normal prostate.

MHC class I antigens are expressed on almost all human nucleated cells and play a vital part in the anti-viral and anti-tumour immune response through their ability to present intra-cellular protein-derived peptides to antigen-specific cytotoxic T lymphocytes (CTLs). In many cancers, including prostate cancer, there is a dramatic loss of MHC class I antigen with tumour progression and 100% of prostate metastases have no class I expressing cells. Also, in one study, expression of class 1 protein, corresponding to an HLA-A genotype has been shown to be partially or completely lost in approximately 90% of the tumours examined: However, only 8% of these patients also had a deletion of the HLA-A1 and HLA-A2 alleles – so that the loss of expression is mostly at the translational level. Up-regulation of expression of MHC class I protein on the cell surface is possible with some immunotherapeutic, chemotherapeutic and radiotherapy regimens. For example, interferon gamma up-regulates MHC class I expression on prostate cancer TRAMP-C1 MHC class I negative tumours. Radiotherapy up-regulates a number of cell surface molecules, including MHC class I and FAS (CD95) that makes tumour cells more susceptible to T-cell-mediated immune attack. Chemotherapeutic drugs such as 5-Aza-2′-deoxycitidine also increase the expression of class I on a number of tumour cell lines, including those of prostate cancer.

Tumour cells, including those in the prostate, can also be eliminated by their lack of expression of MHC class I antigens which are monitored by NK cells through the missing self-hypothesis. However, this hypothesis has also been modified on the discovery of families of inhibitory receptors on NK cells and their corresponding ligands on tumour cells. Such families of receptors including the KIR and LILR receptors (which were originally discovered in myeloid cell populations such as monocytes and Dendritic cells) and their ligands including non-classical MHC molecules such as HLA-G and HLA-E can promote potent immunosuppressive functions, and tumour cells commonly express these ligands in prostate cancer.

Immunotherapy strategies

Cell-based immunotherapy

The concept of cell-based immunotherapy is to expose a whole tumour cell to the immune system to evoke a response to multiple antigens, thus acting as a vaccine. The allogeneic tumour cells are introduced into the patient where these cells can attract antigen presenting cells (APCs) to the site of introduction. The introduced cells are destroyed and taken up by APCs; which present the antigen to T-cells and activate T-cell cytotoxic activity towards tumour cells in the patient. Dranoff et al. examined the immunogenicity of irradiated melanoma cells in mouse models. Retroviral gene transfer of some cytokines into the tumour cells was used to enhance the immunogenicity of the tumour cells. Irradiated transduced vaccine tumour cells were injected. A high level of CD4+ andCD8+ T-cell immune responses was observed. The GM-CSF attracts antigen-presenting cells to the injection site. Other cytokines did not show similar anti-tumour activity. The treatment works by recruiting antigen-presenting cells (APC) such as dendritic cells to injection sites. The vaccine cells are lysed and the debris are taken up by APC, resulting in TH1 and TH2 cell activation which activates cytotoxic cell tumour lysis.

The whole cell allogeneic immunotherapy treatment has been developed further and has used prostate cancer cell lines including the hormone sensitive cell line LNCaP and hormone resistant cell line PC3. In a Phase II trial studying the effect of this type of treatment, dendritic cells and macrophages in addition to eosinophils were present at the site of the intradermal injection, confirming the ability of the transduced cells to secrete GM-CSF *in vivo*. Several patients mounted LNCaP and PC3 reactive antibodies. There is a possible correlation between the antibody titre and time from vaccination. This treatment strategy exposes multiple tumour antigens to potentiate the anti-tumour immune response.

Antigen-specific approach

This strategy focuses on one antigen to evoke an anti-tumour immune response. Various tumour-associated antigens (TAA) antigens have been studied for this type of treatment. Three of them have been targeted. Prostatic-specific antigen (PSA) is a glycoprotein and a serine protease enzyme secreted by the epithelial cells of the prostate gland. Another antigen is prostate acid phosphatase (PAP), which is expressed in the vast majority of prostate cancer cells. The third antigen is the prostate-specific membrane antigen (PSMA). The selected antigen can be carried and introduced to its target using various mechanisms, including a virus vector or DNA plasmid or using one of the host own antigen presenting cell as a vehicle. These methods are discussed in more detail below.

Virus-based vectors

This approach uses a vaccine as a vehicle for the targeted antigen. The most commonly used vector is Vaccinia virus as prime vaccine and fowlpox virus as the booster vaccine (ProstVac VF). This vaccine has a DNA plasmid encoding PSA, in addition to co-stimulatory molecules (lymphocyte function-associated antigen 3 LFA3, CD80 and intracellular adhesion molecule 1 (ICAM1)). All three molecules form the Triad of Costimulatory Molecules (TRICOM) and are designed to synergistically enhance T-cell proliferation. The viral vector is injected intradermally infecting epithelial cells which eventually die with a cell debris including the PSA as antigen, which is taken up by antigen-presenting cells (APC) that present it to CD4+ and CD8+, sensitising it against PSA-producing prostate cancer cells. The immune response can be limited by antibody responses to the viral protein rather than the encoded antigen. This type of treatment is effective if cancer is caused by viruses (HBV, HPV) as the vaccine would be used as a preventive measure.

Virus-based vaccine strategy is limited to narrow virus options that can be used, in addition there is the need for a repeated booster dose. The immune response can be dual in effect: one against the viral vector which is the undesirable but sometime inevitable response and the other against the target antigen carried in the vector virus which is the desirable response. Plasmid DNA-based vaccines aim to avoid the disadvantages of having a carrier viral vector and use plasmid to carry the genetic code for the desired antigen to generate an antigen-specific T-cell response. A plasmid vector is used to encode an antigen sequence, usually a PAP code, and this is injected intradermally with or without GM-CSF to elicit the desired immune response.

APC loaded Ag

In this type of approach, the antigen is loaded onto autologous APC. A recent Food and Drug Administration (FDA) approved treatment

(Sipuleucel-T, Dendreon) is composed of autologous APCs which are loaded with PAP fused with GM-CSF. This fusion protein is called PA2024 and is designed to help with antigen presentation by up-regulating co-stimulatory molecules. The treatment starts by isolating the patient's dentritic cells (DC) by leukapheresis. Then the cells are incubated with the fusion protein for 40 hours. The cells take up the protein. The product is then injected intravenously into the patient. GM-CSF mediates PAP presentation. The elicited immune response includes activation of CD4+ and CD8+.

Monoclonal antibodies

The preferred antigen for this type of approach is PSMA, which is a transmembrane glycoprotein. It has an internalisation motif which makes it an ideal target for monoclonal antibodies. An anti-PSMA antibody has been developed in the mouse and is de-immunised (J591). The antibody is labelled with a radioisotope ^{177}Lutetium. The antibody aims to bind the target prostate cancer cells where the radioisotope Gamma emissions induce cell death.

Immune pathway targeted treatment

This method targets the immune system rather than the tumour. One goal is a feedback molecule. Cytotoxic T Lymphocyte Antigen 4 (CTLA-4) is expressed on the activated T-Cell. It modulates and inhibits T-cell activation, forming a sort of feedback control. It acts as an inhibitor to T-cell activity. The deficiency of CTLA-4 results in lymphoproliferative disorders and the immunosuppressive function of Tregs depends on CTLA-4. The inhibitory activity of CTLA-4 helps tumour tolerance; thus blocking CTLA-4 activity may result in anti-tumour immune activation. A monoclonal antibody (MDX-010 Ipilimumab) modality has been developed which aims at inhibiting Tregs' activity and potentiating CD4+, or CD8+ activity.

Conventional treatment and immunology

Conventional prostate cancer treatment modalities such as hormone, radiotherapy and chemotherapy alter the immune system.

Androgen ablation may boost the anti-tumour immune response. CD4+ number in the prostate gland increases after treatment with anti-androgen, the expansion of naïve T-cells, the increase in effector T-cell response and the production of prostate associated antibodies. All these indicate that androgen deprivation may facilitate a favourable anti-tumour environment. Radiation treatment has a similar effect on the immune system. Hurwitz et al. (2010) found that in 13 prostate cancer patients treated with radiotherapy, there was increased number of CD8+ and NK cells in addition to higher level of Heat Shock Protein (HSP) 27 level. HSP27 acts as immunomodulator and has a role in activatating cytotoxic T cells. Another protein (HMGB1) is released by radiotherapy treated dying cells; Apetoh et al found that HMGB1 is the primary ligand for TLR4 which activates dentritic cells and provoke T cell response. The combination of these conventional treatment modalities with the new immunotherapeutic modalities is being explored in various trials.

Clinical trials in prostate cancer immunotherapy

ProstVAC

Prostatic-specific antigen (PSA) is a target for immunotherapy as it is exclusively expressed in the prostatic epithelial cells. The vaccinia virus elicits humoral and cell-mediated responses and a recombinant form of vaccinia virus encoding PSA (rV-PSA) is used to enhance the immunogenicity of PSA-producing cells and subsequently cell lysis. In a clinical trial of 33 men with prostate cancer recurrence after radical prostatectomy or radiotherapy, rV-PSA was given on three-monthly dose basis. A PSA-specific T cell response was present in five patients in whom PSA blood level stabilised for up to 21 months post treatment. IgG and IgM humoral response was observed in one patient only.

In a Phase II randomised trial, rV-PSA was used in a prime vaccine, with fowlpox virus encoding PSA as a boost vaccine (rF-PSA). Sixty-four patients with organ-confined prostate cancer with biochemical failure after local radical treatment of surgery or radiotherapy were involved in the study. An increase of absolute measure of PSA above 2 ng/ml after surgery or three consecutive increases after radiotherapy constituted biochemical failure. Neoadjuvant chemotherapy or hormonal treatment was given for six months prior to enrolling into the study. All participants had negative bone scans and no evidence of locally advanced disease. Patients were assigned to three treatment arms, one to receive 3rF-PSA vaccine alone, another to receive multiple doses 3rF-PSA vaccine followed by one dose of rV-PSA or to the third arm of multiple doses of rV-PSA followed by a single dose 3rF-PSA. The study did not have a control arm with conventional treatment. The results showed no objective biochemical response, with 45% of patients showing no PSA progression and 78% free of clinical progression at 19 months with no difference between the treatment arms. The immunologic response did not show increases in anti-PSA antibody but there was an increase in PSA-induced T cell proliferation.

Another Phase II trial evaluated the effectiveness of rV-PSA, however, this group used a different T-cell co-stimulatory molecule (B7.1) and IL-2. In addition, a granulocyte-macrophage colony-stimulating factor (GM-CSF) was given to enhance dentritic cell recruitment. This treatment regime was compared to anti-androgen (nilutamide) treatment. A total of 42 hormone refractory metastatic free prostate cancer patients were randomised to receive prime/boost strategy (rV-PSA, rF-PSA), however, the treatment continued rF-PSA boost on a monthly basis until disease recurrence, contrary to the four doses regime in the previous trial. The anti-androgen treatment arm received nilutamide orally on a daily basis until disease recurrence. A cross-over of 12 patients from the vaccine to the anti-androgen arm and eight patients from the anti-androgen to the vaccine arm was observed. There was no difference in time to treatment failure for the vaccine arm (9.9 months) and the nilutamide arm (7.6 months). Time to treatment failure for combined therapy was 13.9 months (vaccine then nilutamide), extending the overall treatment to 25.9 months and 5.2 months (nilutamide then vaccine) with total treatment of 15.9 months. PSA specific T-cell response was observed in varying degrees in the vaccine treatment arm. In the vaccine arm, 13 patients had a decrease in their PSA velocity compared to 16 in the nilutamide arm. It is notable that sequential treatment with hormone following the vaccine showed improved clinical outcome but no conclusion can be drawn, as there is potential selection bias as patients receiving additional treatment had less aggressive disease.

The largest trial to assess PROSTVAC-VF randomised 125 patients from 43 centres in the United States in a 2:1 randomisation ratio to achieve 80% study power. In the vaccine arm, the treatment regime included one priming dose of rV-PSA-TRICOM and six boosts of rF-PSA-TRICOM in addition to GM-CSF adjunct treatment. The control arm received an empty vaccinia vector and an empty fowlpox vector boosts in an identical regime to the treatment arm. Patients who had minimally symptomatic castration-resistant metastatic prostate cancer (mCRPC) were eligible for the study. Progression free survival was similar in both arms, however, at three years the overall survival for the treatment group was better (30%) compared to the control group (17%) lengthening the survival by 8.5 months. The immunological studies did not detect humoral response to PSA vaccine. This well-designed study failed to find a correlation between treatment arm and progression. However, clinically, it did show the improvement in overall survival in the relatively small group of patients.

DNA vaccine

A dose-escalating trial assessing the toxicity of pTVG-HP, a plasmid DNA encoding prostate acid phosphatase (PAP), has been conducted. Twenty-two patients were treated with an escalating dose of intradermal injection of the vaccine with GM-CSF as adjuvant treatment for 6 times over a 14-days interval. The trial confirmed treatment safety. Some 14% of patients developed PAP-specific IFNγ secreting CD8+ T-cells. There was no significant clinical response, however, PSA doubling time was increased in some patients.

GVAX

The GVAX platform involves injecting tumour cells to provoke an immune response, thus presenting to the immune system a cocktail of antigens, which increases the likelihood of a tumour-specific immune response. The tumour cells are genetically modified to secrete GM-CSF. Two cultured allogenic prostate cancer cell lines are used, PC3 and LNCaP. Cell lines are genetically modified to encode the GM-CSF gene and are irradiated to prevent proliferation.

The initial dose-escalating study recruited 80 hormone refractory metastatic prostate cancer patients. Symptomatic patients were excluded from the study. Five dose levels were used. Patients were divided into three different groups: low-dose, moderate-dose and high-dose groups. Treatment ranged from once every 28, 14 days, and it lasted for 6 months, doses started at 100×10^6 cells. The study was stopped prematurely due to disease progression in 90% of patients in addition to adverse events in 2%. However, it did record that the antibody response was proportional to the dose, and was highest for the high-dose group (89%) and lowest for the low-dose group (43%). The median survival was 35 months (high-dose), 20 months (moderate-dose) and 23 months (low-dose) groups, respectively. PSA stabilised in 19% of patients. The study could not determine a maximum tolerable dose.

In Phase III trial by the same group, GVAX was compared to docetaxel and prednisolone treatment for castrate-resistant metastatic prostate cancer patients. Some 626 patients were recruited from more than 100 centres in North America and Europe. GVAX was given in 13 doses every two weeks and then as maintenance doses for a total of six months. The study was prematurely terminated as it showed the futility of achieving the primary end point of superiority in overall survival. The survival analysis showed no superiority in survival of GVAX over the chemotherapy arm.

Another Phase III trial comparing GVAX in combination with docetaxel with patients in the control arm received docetaxel and prednisolone. The study aimed to recruit 600 castrate-resistant prostate cancer patients, however, it was terminated following recruiting only 408 patients due to the high death rate in the treatment arm and the survival advantage in the control arm.

Monoclonal antibody
Ipilimumab

A Phase III double-blind randomised controlled trial compared Ipilimumab to placebo, in castrate-resistant metastatic prostate cancer patients who are receiving radiotherapy. The study by Bristol Myers Squibb is ongoing and aims at recruiting 800 patients and is expected to conclude in 2012 (Trial number NCT00861614).

Radioisotope Ab

A Phase I study looked at anti-prostate specific membrane antigen (PSMA) which was a murine deimmunised antibody (J591). It was attached to the radiometal ^{177}Lu (Lutetium-177). This study recruited 35 castrate-resistant prostate cancer patients. All received the treatment up to three doses. The results showed that myelo-suppression occurred with higher doses. There was no anti-J591 antibody development and all sites of metastasis took up the radio-labelled antibody. PSA stabilisation was observed in almost half of the patients. This study confirmed the excellent targeting ability of anti-PSMA.

A Phase II randomised trial by Weil Cornell University is ongoing and is recruiting 140 patients into two arms. A monoclonal anti PSMA (Murine deimmunised J591) labelled with ^{177}Lu is being used in the treatment arm, and ^{111}In-J591 is being used in the control arm. ^{111}In is a weak radioactive label that does not kill cancer cells. The study is recruiting patients who have been previously treated with surgery or radiotherapy and have biochemical recurrence but not metastasis (NCT00859781).

Another trial by the same group is assessing the suitability of monoclonal antibody treatment of ^{177}Lu-J591 and is recruiting patients with castrate-resistant metastatic prostate cancer (NCT00195039).

A third trial is assessing the toxicity of radio-labelled monoclonal anti-PSMA treatment in combination with docetaxel. Castrate-resistant metastatic prostate cancer patients are being recruited (NCT00916123).

Sipuleucel-T

This is a Phase III trial that recruited 127 patients with 2:1 randomisation ratio of treatment versus placebo. Eligible patients had metastatic prostate cancer with prognosis of no more than three months. The treatment arm patients were given APC8015 (sipuleucel-T) in three doses two weeks apart for each dose. There was 48 hours between the time of apheresis and infusion of treatment product. Placebo group received non-pulsed APCs. Results showed a significant median survival of 25.9 months for the treatment arm compared to 21.4 months for placebo, a total of 4.5 months improvement in survival. In addition, there was an eight-fold increase in T-cell stimulation in the treatment arm.

In an updated survival results of randomised trial comparing three different doses of sipuleucel-T to placebo, the same group recruited 512 castrate-resistant metastatic prostate cancer patients in 2:1, treatment: placebo ratio. The results confirmed the previous trial result of survival benefit for the treatment arm of 25.8 months compared to 21.7 of placebo group. The treatment was generally well tolerated.

Conclusion

The prostate may not look ideal for a naturally effective anti-tumour immune response, but the new emerging evidence links chronic inflammation and cancer development. Chronic prostatitis and HGPIN are pre-cancerous lesions and more research into the immune homeostasis in these conditions may hold some keys to an understanding of immune tolerance and cancer formation. The challenge for anti-tumour immune stimulation remains high and to date the only approved treatment for prostate cancer is expensive and has a survival advantage of 4.1 months. It is huge step forward for immunotherapy in prostate cancer but hardly a paradigm shift. Most of the immunotherapy treatment modalities are aimed at end stage prostate cancer or CRPC and certainly there is scope for targeting early disease and perhaps in pre-cancerous conditions.

Further reading

Coussens LM, Werb Z. Inflammation and cancer. *Nature* 2002;**420**(6917): 860–7.

Drake CG. Prostate cancer as a model for tumour immunotherapy. *Nature Reviews Immunology* 2010;**10**(8): 580.

De Marzo A, et al. Inflammation in prostate carcinogenesis. *Nature Reviews Cancer* 2007;**7**(4): 256.

Dunn GP, Old LJ, Schreiber RD. The immunobiology of cancer immuno-surveillance and immunoediting. *Immunity* 2004;**21**:137–48.

Rajarubendra N, Lawrentschuk N, Bolton DM, Klotz L, Davis ID. Prostate cancer immunology - an update for urologists. *BJU Int* 2010, Nov 10 (ahead of pub.).

Trial references

Published trials with reference in the text starting with 'NCT' are available at www.clinicaltrials.gov.

Apetoh L, Ghiringhelli F, Tesniere A, et al. Toll-like receptor 4-dependent contribution of the immune system to anticancer chemotherapy and radiotherapy. *Nat Med* 2007;**13**:1050–9.

Arlen PM, Gulley JL, Todd N, et al. Antiandrogen, vaccine and combination therapy in patients with nonmetastatic hormone refractory prostate cancer. *J Urol* 2005;**174**:539–46.

Bander NH, Milowsky MI, Nanus DM, Kostakoglu L, Vallabhajosula S, Goldsmith SJ. Phase I trial of 177lutetium-labeled J591, a monoclonal antibody to prostate-specific membrane antigen, in patients with androgen-independent prostate cancer. *J Clin Oncol* 2005;**23**:4591–601.

Eder JP, Kantoff PW, Roper K, et al. A phase I trial of a recombinant vaccinia virus expressing prostate-specific antigen in advanced prostate cancer. *Clin Cancer Res* 2000;**6**:1632–8.

Higano CSF, Somer B, Curti B, Petrylak D, Drake CG, Schnell F, Redfern CH, Schrijvers D, Sacks N. A phase III trial of GVAX immunotherapy for prostate cancer versus docetaxel plus prednisone in asymptomatic, castration-resistant prostate cancer (CRPC). 2009 Genitourinary Cancers Symposium, 2009, Florida.

Hurwitz MD, Kaur P, Nagaraja GM, Bausero MA, Manola J, Asea A. Radiation therapy induces circulating serum Hsp72 in patients with prostate cancer. *Radiother Oncol* 2010;**95**:350–8.

Johnson LE, Frye TP, Arnot AR, et al. Safety and immunological efficacy of a prostate cancer plasmid DNA vaccine encoding prostatic acid phosphatase (PAP). *Vaccine* 2006;**24**:293–303.

Johnson LE, Frye TP, Chinnasamy N, Chinnasamy D, McNeel DG. Plasmid DNA vaccine encoding prostatic acid phosphatase is effective in eliciting autologous antigen-specific CD8+ T cells. *Cancer Immunol Immunother* 2007;**56**:885–95.

Kantoff PW, Higano CS, Shore ND, et al. Sipuleucel-T immunotherapy for castration-resistant prostate cancer. *N Engl J Med* 2010;**363**:411–22.

Kantoff PW, Schuetz TJ, Blumenstein BA, et al. Overall survival analysis of a phase II randomized controlled trial of a Poxviral-based PSA-targeted immunotherapy in metastatic castration-resistant prostate cancer. *J Clin Oncol* 2010;**28**:1099–105.

Kaufman HL, Wang W, Manola J, et al. Phase II randomized study of vaccine treatment of advanced prostate cancer (E7897): A trial of the Eastern Cooperative Oncology Group. *J Clin Oncol* 2004;**22**:2122–32.

McNeel DG, Dunphy EJ, Davies JG, et al. Safety and immunological efficacy of a DNA vaccine encoding prostatic acid phosphatase in patients with stage D0 prostate cancer. *J Clin Oncol* 2009;**27**:4047–54.

Milowsky MI, Nanus DM, Kostakoglu L, Vallabhajosula S, Goldsmith SJ, Bander NH. Phase I trial of yttrium-90-labeled anti-prostate-specific membrane antigen monoclonal antibody J591 for androgen-independent prostate cancer. *J Clin Oncol* 2004;**22**:2522–31.

Small EJ, Schellhammer PF, Higano CS, et al. Placebo-controlled phase III trial of immunologic therapy with sipuleucel-T (APC8015) in patients with metastatic, asymptomatic hormone refractory prostate cancer. *J Clin Oncol* 2006;**24**:3089–94.

Small EJD T, Gerristen WR, Rolland F, Hoskin F, Smith DC, Parker D, Chondros J, Ma J, Hege K. A phase III trial of GVAX immunotherapy for prostate cancer in combination with docetaxel versus docetaxel plus prednisone in symptomatic, castration-resistant prostate cancer (CRPC). 2009 Genitourinary Cancer Symposium. 2009; Florida.

CHAPTER 18

New Approaches to Prostate Cancer

Megan S. Schober[1], *Roger S. Kirby*[2] and *Prokar Dasgupta*[3]

[1]Department of Urology, William Beaumont School of Medicine at Oakland University, Royal Oak, MI, USA
[2]The Prostate Centre, London, UK
[3]Department of Urology, King's College London, Guy's and St Thomas' Hospital NHS Foundation Trust, London, UK

OVERVIEW

- Ablative focal therapy can be useful in low grade localised prostate cancer
- Novel ablative therapies include cryotherapy, stereotactic radiotherapy and high intensity focused ultrasound
- Abiraterone is a novel hormonal treatment for advanced castrate-resistant prostate cancer
- Immunotherapy is an emerging treatment option for castrate-resistant prostate cancer

---

New approaches to prostate cancer

Novel therapies in prostate cancer are being developed for the treatment of both advanced and localised disease. Important factors in developing novel therapies include limitation of injury to surrounding tissues and organs as well as limiting any spread of tumour cells. New techniques are now being developed in the areas of hormonal drug therapy as well as physical ablation of prostate cancer. The following approaches are currently still under investigation in clinical trials, however, preliminary results are quite promising.

New treatments for localised prostate cancer

Ablative focal therapy for localised prostate cancer

Focal therapy for low-risk localised prostate cancer is an option that is gaining popularity. The idea of limiting erectile dysfunction and urinary symptoms by treating only part of the prostate gland is attractive to both clinicians and patients. Techniques that have been tested in whole gland treatments such as HIFU and cryotherapy are now being tested for their efficacy as focal treatments. The clinician utilising these treatment options must bear in mind, however, that at this time diagnostic testing for prostate cancer is not specific enough to rule out multifocal disease in all cases. This means that

ABC of Prostate Cancer, First Edition.
Edited by Prokar Dasgupta and Roger S. Kirby.
© 2012 Blackwell Publishing Ltd. Published 2012 by Blackwell Publishing Ltd.

while an index lesion may be successfully treated by focal therapy, secondary lesions must also be considered.

Focal high intensity focused ultrasound

High intensity focused ultrasound (HIFU) is an emerging treatment that has been demonstrated to be efficacious in treating prostate cancer in multiple studies utilising whole gland treatment. The beam is focused through a trans-rectal ultrasound probe and is able to heat the prostatic tissue between 60 and 100°C, thus destroying the tissue by coagulative necrosis. Although most commonly used as a whole gland treatment, there is some limited data demonstrating its use as a focal treatment. Whole gland treatment studies have consistently demonstrated post-treatment continence rates above 90% and erectile function maintained in 20–46% of patients. A single institution study of 29 patients by Muto et al. (2008) demonstrated 89% and 76% negative biopsy rates at 6 and 12 months respectively with 100% continence. All patients had unilateral, low-risk disease and the method of ablation used in this study consisted of a posterior 'hockey stick' approach. There are currently multiple ongoing clinical trials of focal HIFU treatment in localised, locally recurrent prostate cancer, as well as focal HIFU after radiation failure. Transurethral ultrasonic ablation of the prostate is another technique that is being studied in conjunction with real-time MRI mapping of the prostate. Initial feasibility studies in five patients have demonstrated precise temperature control, reduced treatment times, and theoretic elimination of rectal injuries that may occur during trans-rectal approaches of ultrasonic ablation. Because this study was performed with the sole intent of feasibility, the clinical outcomes of this method are not yet known.

Focal cryotherapy

Cryotherapy of the prostate is a technique that has been used in the whole gland treatment of prostate cancer, especially in the setting of recurrence after radiation of the prostate. It is performed by placing fine needles into the prostate through the perineum while imaging the prostate with trans-rectal ultrasound. The needles are cooled by argon gas so that prostate tissues reach a temperature of −140°C. The needles are then warmed by helium gas. Cell death in the prostate is achieved by ice crystal formation within the cells which destroys cellular architecture. Recent technical innovations in the field prostate cryoablation are making targeted ablation a viable option. In a recent small study of focal cryoablation by Onik et al., 94% of patients maintained a stable PSA with no local recurrences documented by biopsy. All of the patients in this study maintained urinary continence after treatment and most had satisfactory erectile function post-treatment. At this time, true focal cryoablation is technically possible, however, recent studies favour hemi-ablation techniques. Maintaining quality of life in terms of potency and urinary continence is still possible with nerve-sparing hemi-ablation, however, the incidence of under-treatment is theoretically lower.

Stereotactic radiotherapy

Intracranial stereotactic radiosurgery has been utilised to treat various brain lesions for many years. More recently, with the development of frameless systems and improved imaging techniques, stereotactic radiosurgery is now being applied to other organs, including the prostate for treatment localised prostate cancer. This technique is known as stereotactic body radiotherapy or SBRT. Clinical trials have shown that radiosurgery is possible in prostate cancer with a reasonable side-effect profile. Delivery of the radiation dose is extremely precise in this method because of 3D positioning and immobilisation of the target. Because of the exact localisation that can be achieved by stereotactic radiotherapy, a higher dose of radiation can be used per fraction as well as fewer numbers of fractions (hypofractionation). It is suggested that damage to normal tissues surrounding the prostate, such as the rectum, is lessened in this technique as compared to conventional radiation therapy. A recent prospective Phase II trial by King et al. with 33 months of median follow-up has demonstrated a 78% PSA nadir of 0.4 mg/dl. During this short follow-up, none of the patients had biochemical failure.

Novel prostate cancer treatments are continually emerging as current techniques evolve. New hormonal drug therapy and selective ablative techniques, although preliminarily promising, are currently being tested in long-term studies to determine their overall survival benefit and efficacy.

New treatments for metastatic prostate cancer

Abiraterone

Abiraterone is a novel hormonal treatment for castrate-resistant prostate cancer (CRPC) that is currently being tested in Phase III clinical trials. It has been demonstrated that even in patients who have undergone androgen ablation therapy or surgical castration, high levels of intratumoral androgens can still be detected. This is due to the ability of prostate tumours to continue to utilise androgen receptor (AR) signalling pathways and over-expression of enzymes important for androgen synthesis. This allows prostate tumour cells to convert adrenal androgens to testosterone, thus giving the tumour cells 'fuel' for growth and expansion. Abiraterone was developed with the aim of blocking this pathway of testosterone production. Abiraterone is a selective inhibitor of the cytochrome P (CYP) 17 microsomal enzyme. CYP17 is involved in steroidogenesis in two different pathways. The first mechanism is via its 17α-hydroxylase activity. Pregnenolone is converted to 17OH-pregnenolone by 17α-hydroxylase and subsequently is converted to 11-deoxycortisol and eventually cortisol. The second mechanism of the CYP17 enzyme is via C17,20-lyase. It is this pathway that is important in CRPC progression. C17,20-lyase converts 17OH-pregnenolone to dehydroepiandrosterone (DHEA) which is then converted to androstenedione (Figure 18.1). Androstenedione is converted to testosterone by 17β-hydroxysteroid dehydrogenase. DHEA, androstendione and estradiol are all capable of stimulating the androgen receptor and this is thought to be one of the mechanisms that may lead to failure of traditional anti-androgen treatments.

Ketoconazole is one of the anti-androgen treatments that has the ability to block adrenal androgens through its inhibition of cytochrome P450, however, significant side-effects such as hepatotoxicity, nausea, vomiting and lethargy are relatively common

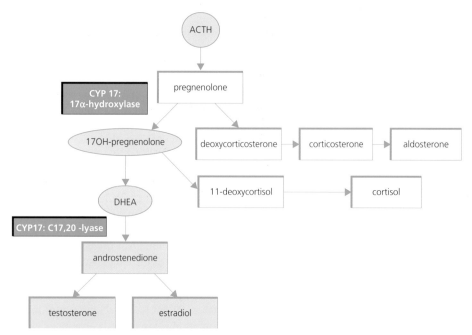

Figure 18.1 The CYP17 enzymes 17 α-hydroxylase and C17, 20-lyase are both irreversibly inhibited by abiraterone. This leads to decreased production of the AR stimulating molecules DHEA, androstenedione, testosterone and estradiol.

with this treatment which limit its use. In abiraterone treatment, ACTH levels were elevated as high as five times normal levels secondary to a negative feedback loop driven by decreased levels of cortisol from the inhibition of 17α-hydroxylase. Side-effects of abiraterone treatment appeared to be due to the increase of ACTH from this negative feedback mechanism. Adverse events included hypokalemia, hypertension and lower extremity edema, but these were all effectively treated during the Phase I trial with the aldosterone antagonist eplerenone. Two other significant side-effects documented during the Phase I trial were migraine headache and asthma exacerbation. The cause of the migraine headache was undetermined, but did resolve with dexamethasone which functions by lowering ACTH levels, therefore it may have been secondary to abiraterone treatment. The patient with the asthma exacerbation was successfully treated with high dose steroids. In a subsequent Phase II trial, the addition of low dose prednisone to abiraterone treatment proved beneficial in limiting most of the side-effects due to mineralacorticoid excess.

PSA decline greater than 50% of pre-treatment values was demonstrated in both Phase I and Phase II trials. In the Phase II study, PSA decline was demonstrated in patients who had received ketoconazole as well as ketoconazole-naive patients. Patients also had objective anti-tumour response by Response Evaluation Criteria in Solid Tumors (RECIST) criteria. The overall median time to PSA progression was 169 days. Patients who had received ketoconazole treatment prior to abiraterone had a median time to progression of 99 days while those who were had not been treated with ketoconazole had median time to progression at 198 days. Interestingly, 69% of patients in the Phase II study had circulating tumour cell counts (CTC) in an unfavourable range prior to abiraterone but 34% of these patients converted to a favourable CTC state after treatment. Abiraterone is a promising new hormonal therapy that appears to have significant benefit in patients with CRPC. Data from Phase I and Phase II trials have successfully demonstrated biochemical, radiologic, and modest clinical benefit from abiraterone treatment. Abiraterone is currently being tested in randomised Phase III clinical trials and the benefit to overall survival will be better determined.

Sipuleucel

Sipuleucel is an immunotherapeutic agent that uses a patient's own immune system to actively target prostate cancer cells. Patients first undergo leukophoresis and the mixed cell population obtained includes antigen-presenting cells (APC) which are cultured *ex vivo* and incubated with a recombinant fusion protein of the antigen PAP and the cytokine granulocyte/macrophage colony stimulating factor (PAP-GM-CSF). PAP is expressed in 95% of prostate cancers and GM-CSF is a leukocyte growth factor. The cells are then infused into the patient three or four days after initial leukophoresis. The vaccine has been tested in three separate randomised, double-blind, placebo-controlled multicentre trials. Results of the IMPACT trial were recently published in the *New England Journal of Medicine* and have demonstrated a median survival benefit of 4.1 months for men treated with sipuleucel versus placebo. The actual time to objective disease progression, however, was not significantly different between placebo and study-treated patient groups. This observation had been previously reported in other trials using sipuleucel and it has been suggested that this is secondary to delayed anti-tumour response after active immunotherapy relative to objective disease progression which occurs early in castrate-resistant prostate cancer patients. Overall, the drug appeared to be well tolerated by patients with the only adverse effects reported being secondary to cytokine release, such as fever, chills, and fatigue. Treatment with sipuleucel did not preclude subsequent treatment and in fact, the majority of patients treated with sipuleucel in the IMPACT trial went on to receive docetaxel. The authors of the study found no evidence that docetaxel treatment confounded the results of the IMPACT trial. An advantage of this drug is that only a single treatment should be necessary.

References

Muto S, Yoshii T, Saito K Kamiyama Y, Ide H, Horie S. Focal therapy with high-intensity-focused ultrasound in the treatment of localized prostate cancer. *Jpn J Clin Oncol* 2008; **38**(3):192–9.

Further reading

Buyyounouski MK, Price Jr. RA, Harris EER, Miller R, Tomé W, Schefter T, et al. Stereotactic body radiotherapy for primary management of early-stage, low- to intermediate-risk prostate cancer: Report of the American Society for Therapeutic Radiology and Oncology Emerging Technology Committee. *Int Radiat Oncol Biol Phys* 2010; **76**:1297–304.

Danila D, Morris M, de Bono JS, Ryan CJ, Denmeade SR, Smith MR, et al. Phase II multicenter study of abiraterone acetate plus prednisone therapy in patients with docetaxal-treated castration-resistant prostate cancer. *J Clin Onc* 2010; **28**(9):1496–501.

Kantoff PW, Higano CS, Shore ND, Berger ER, Small EJ, Penson DF, et al. Sipuleucel-T immunotherapy for castration-resistant prostate cancer. *N Engl J Med* 2010: **353**:411–22.

Mouraviev V, Johansen TEB, Polascik TJ. Contemporary results of focal therapy for prostate cancer using cryoablation. *J Endourol* 2010; **24**(5):827–34.

Siddiqui K, Chopra R, Vedula S, Sugar L, Haider M, Boyes A, et al. MRI-guided transurethral ultrasound therapy of the prostate gland using real-time thermal mapping: initial studies. *Urology* 2010 Aug. In press.

Index